Medical-Surgical Nursing Certification Practice Q&A

Medical-Surgical Nursing Certification Practice Q&A

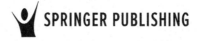 SPRINGER PUBLISHING

Springer Publishing Company, LLC
11 West 42nd Street, New York, NY 10036
www.springerpub.com

Acquisitions Editor: Elizabeth Nieginski
Compositor: diacriTech
ISBN: 9780826146014
ebook ISBN: 9780826146021
DOI: 10.1891/9780826146021

22 23 24 25 / 5 4 3 2 1

The author and the publisher of this Work have made every effort to use sources believed to be reliable to provide information that is accurate and compatible with the standards generally accepted at the time of publication. The author and publisher shall not be liable for any special, consequential, or exemplary damages resulting, in whole or in part, from the readers' use of, or reliance on, the information contained in this book. The publisher has no responsibility for the persistence or accuracy of URLs for external or third-party Internet websites referred to in this publication and does not guarantee that any content on such websites is, or will remain, accurate or appropriate.

Library of Congress Cataloging-in-Publication Data

LCCN: 2022939580

Contact sales@springerpub.com to receive discount rates on bulk purchases.

Publisher's Note: **New and used products purchased from third-party sellers are not guaranteed for quality, authenticity, or access to any included digital components.**

Printed in the United States of America by Hatteras, Inc.

Contents

Preface

Welcome to *Medical-Surgical Nursing Certification Practice Q&A*! Congratulations on taking this important step on your journey to becoming a certified medical-surgical nurse. This resource is based on the most recent blueprints for the Certified Medical-Surgical Registered Nurse (CMSRN®) examination and the Medical-Surgical Nursing Certification (MEDSURG-BC™) examination and was developed by experienced medical-surgical nurses. It is designed to help you sharpen your specialty knowledge with 300 practice questions organized by body system, as well as strengthen your knowledge-application and test-taking skills with two 150-question practice exams. It also includes essential information about the CMSRN® and MEDSURG-BC™ examinations, including eligibility requirements, exam content subject areas and question distributions, and tips for successful exam preparation.

▶ PART I: PRACTICE QUESTIONS

Part I includes 11 chapters based on body system: Gastrointestinal System; Pulmonary System; Cardiovascular System; Hematological System; Endocrine System; Immune System; Urinary System; Musculoskeletal System; Neurological System; Eyes, Ears, Nose, and Throat; and Integumentary System. Each chapter includes high-quality, exam-style questions and comprehensive answers with rationales that address both correct and incorrect answers. Part I is designed to strengthen your specialty knowledge and is formatted for ultimate studying convenience—answer the questions on each page and simply turn the page for the corresponding answers and rationales. No need to refer to the back of the book for the answers.

▶ PART II: PRACTICE EXAMS

Part II includes two 150-question practice exams that align with the exam content subject areas and question distributions found on the most recent blueprints for the CMSRN® and MEDSURG-BC™ examinations. These practice exams are designed to help you strengthen your knowledge-application and test-taking skills. Maximize your preparation and simulate the exam experience by setting aside 3 hours to complete one practice exam. Comprehensive answers and rationales that address both correct and incorrect answers are located in the chapters immediately following the practice exams.

   We know life is busy, and being able to prepare for your exam efficiently and effectively is paramount. This resource gives you the tools and confidence you need to succeed. For additional exam preparation resources, including self-paced online courses, online QBanks, comprehensive review texts, and high-yield study guides, visit www.springerpub.com/examprep. Best of luck to you on your certification journey!

Introduction: Medical-Surgical Nursing Certification Exams and Tips for Preparation

▶ MEDICAL-SURGICAL NURSING CERTIFICATION BOARD

ELIGIBILITY REQUIREMENTS

The CMSRN® examination is developed and administered by the Medical-Surgical Nursing Certification Board (MSNCB). To qualify to take the exam, you must meet the following requirements:

- Hold an active, unencumbered RN license in the United States, U.S. territories, or Canada.
- Have 2 years of practice in a medical-surgical setting.
- Have a minimum of 2,000 hours of practice, including clinical, management, or education practice, in a medical-surgical setting in the last 3 years.

Qualified applicants may submit an online application at www.msncb.org. Successful candidates will receive an Authorization to Test and must schedule the exam within a 90-day window. The exam fee is $375; the fee for members of the Academy of Medical-Surgical Nurses (AMSN) is $255. Refer to the MSNCB website for complete eligibility requirements, pricing, and certification information: www.msncb.org.

ABOUT THE EXAMINATION

The CMSRN® examination takes 3 hours and consists of 150 multiple-choice questions with four answer options. You must select the single best answer. Only 125 questions are scored, and the remaining 25 questions are used as pretest questions. It is impossible to know which questions are scored, so be sure to answer all of the questions to the best of your ability. See Table 1 for categories and question distribution. For more detailed exam content information, refer to the CMSRN® exam blueprint at www.msncb.org/medical-surgical/get-certified/exam/exam-blueprint.

Table 1. CMSRN® Exam Categories and Question Distribution

Categories	Percentage of Questions
Gastrointestinal	16%–18%
Pulmonary	15%–17%
Cardiovascular/Hematological	16%–18%
Diabetes (Type 1 and 2)/Other Endocrine/ Immunological	18%–20%

Table 1. CMSRN® Exam Categories and Question Distribution (*continued*)

Categories	Percentage of Questions
Urological/Renal	14%–16%
Musculoskeletal/Neurological/Integumentary	15%–17%

▶ AMERICAN NURSES CREDENTIALING CENTER

ELIGIBILITY REQUIREMENTS

The MEDSURG-BC™ examination is developed and administered by the American Nurses Credentialing Center (ANCC). To qualify to take the exam, you must meet the following requirements:

- Hold an active, unencumbered RN license in a U.S. state or territory or the equivalent legally recognized certification in another country.
- Have 2 years of practice in a medical-surgical setting.
- Have a minimum of 2,000 hours of practice in a medical-surgical setting in the last 3 years.
- Have a minimum of 30 hours of continuing-education credits in medical-surgical nursing within the last 3 years.

Qualified applicants may submit an online application at www.nursingworld.org/our-certifications/medical-surgical-nurse/. Successful candidates will receive an Authorization to Test and must schedule the exam within a 90-day window. The exam fee is $395; the fee for members of the American Nurses Association (ANA) is $295. Refer to the ANCC website for complete eligibility requirements, pricing, and certification information: www.nursingworld.org.

ABOUT THE EXAMINATION

The MEDSURG-BC™ examination takes 3 hours and consists of 150 multiple-choice questions with four answer options. You must select the single best answer. Only 125 questions are scored, and the remaining 25 questions are used as pretest questions. It is impossible to know which questions are scored, so be sure to answer all of the questions to the best of your ability. See Table 2 for content domains and question distribution. For more detailed exam content information, refer to the MEDSURG-BC™ test content outline at www.nursingworld.org/~499857/globalassets/certification/certification-specialty-pages/resources/test-content-outlines/medsurg-tco-after.pdf.

Table 2. MEDSURG-BC™ Exam Content Domains and Question Distribution

Content Domain	Percentage of Questions
Assessment and Diagnosis	42%
Planning, Implementation, and Evaluation	46%
Professional Role	12%

▶ TIPS FOR EXAM PREPARATION

You know the old joke about how to get to Carnegie Hall—practice, practice, practice! The same is true when seeking certification. Practice and preparation are key to your success on exam day. Here are 10 tips to help you prepare:

1. Allow at least 6 months to fully prepare for the exam. Do not rely on last-minute cramming sessions.
2. Thoroughly review the CMSRN® or MEDSURG-BC™ blueprint so that you know exactly what to expect. Pay close attention to the question topics. Identify your strengths, weaknesses, and knowledge gaps, so you know where to focus your studies. Review all of the supplementary resources available on the CMSRN® or MEDSURG-BC™ website.
3. Create a study timeline with weekly or monthly study tasks. Be as specific as possible—identify *what* you will study, *how* you will study, and *when* you will study.
4. Use several exam-prep resources that provide different benefits. For example, use a comprehensive review to build your specialty knowledge, use this resource and other question banks to strengthen your knowledge-application and test-taking skills, and use a high-yield review to brush up on key concepts in the days leading up to the exam. Springer Publishing offers a wide range of print and online exam-prep products to suit all of your study needs; visit www.springerpub.com/examprep.
5. Assess your level of knowledge and performance on practice questions and exams. Carefully consider why you may be missing certain questions. Continually analyze your strengths, weaknesses, and knowledge gaps, and adjust your study plan accordingly.
6. Minimize distraction as much as possible while you are studying. You will feel more calm, centered, and focused, which will lead to increased knowledge retention.
7. Engage in stress-reducing activities, particularly in the month leading up to the exam. Yoga, stretching, and deep-breathing exercises can be beneficial. If you are feeling frustrated or anxious while studying, take a break. Go for a walk, play with your child or pet, or finish a chore that has been weighing on you. Wait until you feel more refreshed before returning to study.
8. Focus on your health in the weeks and days before the exam. Eat balanced meals, stay hydrated, and minimize alcohol consumption. Get as much sleep as possible, particularly the night before the exam.
9. Eat a light meal before the exam but limit your liquid consumption. The clock does not stop for restroom breaks! Ensure that you know exactly where you are going and how long it will take to get there. Leave with plenty of time to spare to reduce travel-related stress and ensure that you arrive on time.
10. Remind yourself to relax and stay calm. You have prepared, and you know your stuff. Visualize the success that is just ahead of you and make it happen. When you pass, celebrate!

Pass Guarantee

If you use this resource to prepare for your exam and you do not pass, you may return it for a refund of your full purchase price. To receive a refund, you must return your product along with a copy of your original receipt and exam score report. Product must be returned and received within 180 days of the original purchase date. This excludes tax, shipping, and handling. One offer per person and address. Refunds will be issued within 8 weeks from acceptance and approval. This offer is valid for U.S. residents only. Void where prohibited. To initiate a refund, please contact customer service at CS@springerpub.com.

Part I
Practice Questions

Gastrointestinal System

1. A patient with a riboflavin deficiency is experiencing cheilitis. Which of the following would the nurse expect to find during assessment?

   A. A smooth tongue with a red, slick appearance
   B. White, curd-like lesions on the tongue and palate
   C. Inflammation of the lips with fissuring, scaling, and crusting
   D. Recessed gums with purulent pockets

2. A patient is passing large, fatty, frothy, and foul-smelling stools. What other clinical signs may the nurse observe with this symptom?

   A. Abdominal tenderness, weight loss, and jaundice
   B. Tachycardia, intense back pain, and hypertension
   C. Blood in stool, abdominal cramping, and low hemoglobin levels
   D. Alopecia, frequent canker sores, and dry mouth

3. A patient diagnosed with chronic obstructive pulmonary disease (COPD) is malnourished. Which of the following nursing diagnoses outlines the link between COPD and malnutrition?

   A. Imbalanced nutrition of less than body requirements related to decreased food absorption
   B. Self-care deficit (feeding) related to decreased endurance and fatigue
   C. Risk for impaired skin integrity due to poor nutritional state
   D. Deficient fluid volume related to decreased absorption of fluids

4. The nurse is caring for a patient with suspected septicemia who is on total parental nutrition (TPN). Which nursing action helps to provide diagnostic information related to the source of the infection?

   A. Infusing dextrose 10% in water via a peripheral intravenous site while discontinuing the TPN to prevent hypoglycemia
   B. Removing the central venous catheter per healthcare provider order and sending the catheter tip for culture and sensitivity testing
   C. Changing the TPN tubing and filter, then reattaching it to the existing central venous catheter
   D. Asking whether the patient touched or manipulated the catheter site

1. C) Inflammation of the lips with fissuring, scaling, and crusting

Cheilitis is an inflammation of the lips (usually lower) accompanied by fissuring, scaling, or crusting of the lips. It is associated with riboflavin deficiency. A red, smooth tongue with a slick appearance is a sign of a cobalamin deficiency. White, curd-like lesions are associated with candidiasis. Recessed gums with purulent pockets are signs of periodontitis.

2. A) Abdominal tenderness, weight loss, and jaundice

Steatorrhea is the passage of large amounts of fat as fatty, frothy, foul-smelling stool. It may be a sign of chronic pancreatitis, biliary obstruction, or malabsorption problems. The nurse should assess for signs of chronic pancreatitis (fever, abdominal tenderness, weight loss), biliary obstruction (jaundice), or malabsorption (weight loss, diarrhea, pallor, and fatigue). Tachycardia, intense back pain, and hypertension can be associated with abdominal aneurysm. Blood in stool, cramping, and low hemoglobin levels may be present in inflammatory bowel conditions. Alopecia, frequent canker sores, and dry mouth are common in patients undergoing antineoplastic therapy.

3. B) Self-care deficit (feeding) related to decreased endurance and fatigue

COPD often results in malnutrition and low albumin levels in the body. This occurs because the patient experiences respiratory fatigue and decreased endurance and has difficulty eating due to breathing issues. Imbalanced nutrition due to decreased food absorption often occurs in gastrointestinal disorders that affect bowel function. Risk for impaired skin integrity is linked to malnutrition in all patient populations. Deficient fluid volume occurs in dehydration and instances in which patients experience excessive diuresis.

4. B) Removing the central venous catheter per healthcare provider order and sending the catheter tip for culture and sensitivity testing

To diagnose the presence of infection and determine the causative organism, cultures of the catheter tip (if the catheter has been removed) or of the blood in the catheter (if it is still place) are performed. Continuing to infuse fluid through the central line may put the patient at risk. Changing the TPN tubing should occur after a new line is in situ. Asking the patient about touching or manipulating the site doesn't provide a direct way to determine the source and causative organism for the septicemia.

5. The nurse is assessing a male patient for the presence of metabolic syndrome. His fasting blood glucose level is 196 mg/dL (11 mmol/L) and waist circumference is greater than 102 cm. Other diagnostic criteria the nurse should obtain include:

   A. Triglycerides, high-density lipoprotein cholesterol, and blood pressure.
   B. Low-density lipoprotein cholesterol, heart rate, and body mass index (BMI).
   C. Triglycerides, total cholesterol level, and blood pressure.
   D. BMI, total cholesterol, and resting heart rate.

6. A patient who had a bowel resection surgery 4 hours ago is receiving ondansetron 4 mg intravenously every 2 to 4 hours as needed. Which of the following nursing diagnoses apply to this patient?

   A. Nausea related to general anesthetic as evidenced by episodes of nausea and vomiting
   B. Compromised fluid volume related to prolonged vomiting as evidenced by decreased urine output
   C. Nutritional compromise related to nausea and vomiting as evidenced by lack of interest in eating
   D. Imbalanced nutrition due to nothing-by-mouth status prior to surgery

7. A patient who smokes 24 cigarettes a day has stomatitis. What would the nurse expect to find during assessment?

   A. Painful ulcers of the mouth and lips
   B. Inflamed gingivae and bleeding during toothbrushing
   C. Pain and swelling of the parotid gland
   D. Excessive salivation, halitosis, and sore mouth

8. A patient is admitted with a gastrointestinal bleed of unknown origin. Which diagnostic test would be recommended for this patient?

   A. Abdominal ultrasonography
   B. CT
   C. MRI
   D. Barium enema

9. What is the most common concurrent diagnosis with gastroesophageal reflux disorder (GERD) that puts a patient at an increased risk for cancer?

   A. Barrett's esophagus
   B. Esophagitis
   C. Vincent's infection
   D. *Helicobacter pylori* infection

10. A patient returns to the medical unit after a colonoscopy. Which of the following symptoms would result in the nurse calling the healthcare provider immediately?

    A. Abdominal cramping
    B. Abdominal distension and tenesmus
    C. Presence of watery stool
    D. Shoulder pain and discomfort

(See answers next page.)

5. A) Triglycerides, high-density lipoprotein cholesterol, and blood pressure.
The additional diagnostic criteria for metabolic syndrome include triglycerides greater than 150 mg/dL (1.7 mmol/L) or drug treatment for elevated triglycerides, high-density lipoprotein cholesterol greater than 34 mg/dL (0.9 mmol/L) in men, and blood pressure greater than 130 mmHg systolic or 85 mmHg diastolic.

6. A) Nausea related to general anesthetic as evidenced by episodes of nausea and vomiting
Postoperative nausea and vomiting are most commonly linked to the use of general anesthesia during surgery. Ondansetron is given to decrease episodes of nausea and vomiting by acting on the chemotherapy trigger zone in the brain. Decreased urine output may be related to the surgical procedure and blood or general fluid loss. The patient does not show a lack of interest in eating, having just had a surgical procedure. The patient has had restricted food intake for less than 24 hours and will receive fluid in the preoperative, intraoperative, and postoperative periods.

7. D) Excessive salivation, halitosis, and sore mouth
Stomatitis is an inflammation of the mouth. It can result from trauma; pathogens; smoking; or renal, liver, and hematologic diseases. It is also associated with chemotherapy drugs and radiation. Clinical manifestations include excessive salivation, halitosis, and sore mouth. Aphthous stomatitis (canker sore) is a painful ulcer of the mouth and lips. Gingivitis is inflamed gingivae that bleed during toothbrushing. Parotitis is an inflammation of the parotid gland usually caused by *Staphylococcus* bacteria.

8. C) MRI
An MRI is noninvasive imaging using radiofrequency waves and a magnetic field. This procedure is used to detect hepatic metastases and sources of gastrointestinal (GI) bleeding and to stage colorectal cancer. An abdominal ultrasound helps to study abdominal masses and assess ascites. A CT detects biliary tract, liver, and pancreatic disorders. Use of contrast helps with better visualization of structures. A barium enema contains a contrast medium; it is administered rectally and then x-rayed. It helps to screen for structural abnormalities of the GI tract.

9. A) Barrett's esophagus
Barrett's esophagus is considered a precancerous lesion and places the patient at risk for esophageal cancer. Esophagitis is an inflammation of the esophagus. Vincent's infection is acute necrotizing ulcerative gingivitis due to poor oral hygiene and nutritional deficiency of B and C vitamins. *Helicobacter pylori* infection is related to the development of ulcers in the gastrointestinal tract.

10. B) Abdominal distension and tenesmus
The most significant complication of a colonoscopy is bowel perforation. This manifests as rectal bleeding, abdominal distension, and tenesmus (cramping rectal pain). Abdominal cramping is an expected side effect of a colonoscopy. Liquid stool is expected secondary to the preoperative bowel prep. Laparoscopy, not colonoscopy, results in shoulder pain and discomfort due to retained carbon dioxide from the procedure.

11. The healthcare provider orders a "step-down" approach for the management of gastroesophageal reflux disorder. Which nursing statement best describes this approach to this type of pharmacologic management?

    A. "You will start by taking a proton pump inhibitor medication and then slowly titrate down to prescription histamine H_2 receptor drugs and then antacids."

    B. "You will focus your drug therapy on antacids and over-the-counter histamine H_2 receptor blocking agents."

    C. "You will start by taking antacid medication and then move to histamine H_2 receptor blockers, then to proton pump inhibitors."

    D. "This approach includes the use of prokinetic drug therapy and cholinergic drugs."

12. A patient with suspected esophageal cancer asks the nurse why a bronchoscopy has been ordered. What should the nurse teach the patient regarding the purpose of this diagnostic test?

    A. "This examination can help detect whether there is any malignant involvement in your lungs."

    B. "This is an important tool to stage esophageal cancer."

    C. "This test assesses the vital capacity of your lungs."

    D. "This test will help make a definitive diagnosis of malignancy in the esophagus."

13. A patient is admitted to the medical unit with a diagnosis of gastritis. What should the nurse assess for in the patient's history?

    A. Use of cimetidine

    B. Use of antacid therapy

    C. History of pantoprazole use

    D. Nonsteroidal anti-inflammatory drug use

14. A patient with an upper gastrointestinal bleed is prescribed a continuous intravenous infusion of octreotide. The nurse should teach the patient:

    A. "This drug decreases the amount of hydrochloric acid in your stomach by releasing a hormone called *gastrin*. This allows the site of the bleed to heal."

    B. "This drug causes vasocontraction and smooth muscle activity of your gastrointestinal tract. It reduces the pressure in the blood vessels surrounding your liver."

    C. "This drug neutralizes acid and maintains gastric pH in a more alkalotic environment. It helps to heal gastric ulcers."

    D. "This drug inhibits the cellular pump in your stomach responsible for the production of hydrochloric acid."

15. A patient is admitted for preoperative care for gastric cancer. The patient is in poor physical condition and has a low serum albumin level. Which of these nursing interventions is the most appropriate at this time?

    A. Asking the patient about their level of coping with their diagnosis

    B. Completing patient teaching regarding the surgery

    C. Problem-solving strategies to help increase the patient's food intake

    D. Ensuring that the patient is taking a clear fluid diet to rest the bowel before surgery

(See answers next page.)

11. A) "You will start by taking a proton pump inhibitor medication and then slowly titrate down to prescription histamine H$_2$ receptor drugs and then antacids."
There are two approaches to drug therapy to treat gastroesophageal reflux disorder: step-up and step-down approach. The step-down approach starts with proton pump inhibitors and titrates down to prescription histamine H$_2$ blockers and then antacids. A step-up approach starts with antacid therapy, moves to histamine H$_2$ receptor blockers, and then to proton pump inhibitors. Prokinetic drug therapy is used to move food through the gastrointestinal tract faster and cholinergic drugs help to quicken gastric emptying. However, these medications are used as adjuncts to standard therapy.

12. A) "This examination can help detect whether there is any malignant involvement in your lungs."
The purpose of a bronchoscopy for a patient with suspected esophageal cancer is to determine whether there is any suspected malignancy in the lungs. A pulmonary function test assesses lung capacity and function. An endoscopic ultrasound is used to stage esophageal cancer. CT scanning and MRI are also used to assess the extent of disease. Endoscopy with biopsy is necessary to make a definitive diagnosis of malignancy in the esophagus.

13. D) Nonsteroidal anti-inflammatory drug use
Eliminating the cause is what is needed to treat acute gastritis. Nonsteroidal anti-inflammatory drugs, corticosteroids, and salicylates are common medications causing this condition. Antacid therapy, pantoprazole, and cimetidine are used to treat it.

14. A) "This drug decreases the amount of hydrochloric acid in your stomach by releasing a hormone called *gastrin*. This allows the site of the bleed to heal."
Octreotide (Sandostatin) is used for upper gastrointestinal bleeding and esophageal varices. It decreases splanchnic blood flow and hydrochloric acid secretion by decreasing gastrin. Vasopressin causes vasoconstriction and reduces portal hypertension. Antacid medications reduce gastric pH and heal ulcers. Proton pump inhibitors (e.g., omeprazole) inhibit the cellular pump, which is necessary for hydrochloric acid secretion.

15. C) Problem-solving strategies to help increase the patient's food intake
Surgery will be delayed until the patient becomes more physically able to withstand the surgery. A positive nutritional state enhances wound healing as well as the ability to withstand infection. A low albumin level is a clinical indicator for malnutrition. The nurse is required to help ready the patient for surgery, and although emotional support is important, the other interventions are aimed at improving the patient's physical condition. It would not be appropriate to teach about the surgery at this time because the patient needs to be physically able to have surgery. Bowel rest is not required preoperatively.

16. A patient is admitted to the hospital for *Escherichia coli* food poisoning. Which intervention should the nurse expect to implement first?

    A. Initiate antibiotic therapy.
    B. Initiate supportive care to maintain intravascular volume.
    C. Isolate the food source for the infection.
    D. Provide antiemetic therapy for vomiting.

17. The nurse notes that three patients on the medical unit had sudden episodes of explosive, watery diarrhea accompanied by nausea and vomiting. Which of the following pathogens is the most likely source of this acute infection?

    A. Norovirus
    B. *Clostridium difficile*
    C. *Cryptosporidium*
    D. *Salmonella*

18. A patient has had severe diarrhea of an unknown origin for 3 days. Which nursing assessment is the highest priority for this patient?

    A. Assess serum sodium levels.
    B. Assess for potassium losses.
    C. Weigh the patient daily.
    D. Assess urea and creatinine levels.

19. A patient with advanced dementia is experiencing fecal incontinence. Which nursing intervention will help to promote dignity for the patient?

    A. Request that the patient have a private room and commode at the bedside.
    B. Ensure that the patient's undergarments are changed immediately after incontinence.
    C. Create a bowel routine based on the patient's regular bowel patterns.
    D. Insert a rectal tube to help facilitate the removal of stool.

20. An adolescent patient is experiencing severe constipation. Which question helps the nurse to understand factors potentially contributing to this problem?

    A. "Do you drink soda, energy drinks, or juice on a regular basis?"
    B. "Does anyone in your family have a history of chronic constipation?"
    C. "How long does it take you to have a bowel movement once you sit on the toilet?"
    D. "Are you comfortable defecating while at school, or do you hold it until you get home?"

21. A patient develops acute abdominal pain of an unknown origin. He has abdominal rigidity and is on oxygen therapy. What is the priority intervention?

    A. Increase the flow rate of the oxygen.
    B. Initiate intravenous (IV) access with two large-bore IV catheters.
    C. Obtain blood for a complete blood count and serum electrolyte panel.
    D. Insert a nasogastric tube.

(See answers next page.)

16. B) Initiate supportive care to maintain intravascular volume.
Escherichia coli food poisoning can cause intravascular fluid loss, so supportive care should be initiated to maintain intravascular volume. Antibiotic therapy for this condition is controversial. Isolating the food source for contamination will not help with acute treatment. Administration of medications, such as antiemetics, would not be the initial priority.

17. A) Norovirus
The symptoms are consistent with norovirus, which is manifested by explosive, watery diarrhea; nausea; vomiting; and abdominal cramps. It moves quickly between patients and outbreaks are common in institutional settings. *Clostridium difficile* is usually associated with antibiotic treatment and is contagious between patients. Fever, leukocytosis, and strong-smelling watery stools are the most common symptoms. Salmonella is associated with nausea, vomiting, fever, chills, muscle pain, and joint pain. Cryptosporidium is characterized by a persistent cough, watery diarrhea, lack of appetite, stomach pain/cramps, and nausea/vomiting.

18. B) Assess for potassium losses.
All of these interventions are important. However, the highest priority is to assess potassium losses because they may be severe in this patient. This may lead to cardiac arrhythmias. Sodium levels may be increased due to dehydration. Daily weights may indicate total volume loss. An increase in urea and creatinine may indicate prerenal failure from volume losses.

19. C) Create a bowel routine based on the patient's regular bowel patterns.
The nurse should create a bowel routine based on the patient's regular bowel routine to help prevent incontinence. The patient has dementia and needs to be prompted to defecate; a private room and access to a commode will not help fecal incontinence. Allowing the patient to defecate in the undergarments does not promote dignity. A rectal tube is not an appropriate treatment for this patient.

20. D) "Are you comfortable defecating while at school, or do you hold it until you get home?"
The nurse should think about how the patient's developmental stage may be affecting the development of constipation. The patient may be holding in bowel movements after breakfast and lunch while at school. The nurse should assess for dietary factors, such as fiber intake, rather than sugary beverages such as soda, energy drinks, and juice. A family history would be appropriate if the patient was exhibiting symptoms of gastrointestinal disorders (e.g., Crohn's disease). *Constipation* is defined by the frequency of bowel movements and the appearance of stool, not the time it takes to complete a bowel movement.

21. B) Initiate intravenous (IV) access with two large-bore IV catheters.
Because the origin of the severe abdominal pain is unknown, the nurse should ensure IV access with two large-bore catheters in the event the patient requires fluid boluses. The patient is not demonstrating signs of hypoxia, so the oxygen flow rate can stay the same. A complete blood count and electrolyte panel are appropriate but can be collected during or after the IV is initiated. The insertion of a nasogastric tube may also be appropriate, but the patient requires IV access first.

22. The nurse is evaluating a patient's response to enteral feeding via a jejunostomy. What would the nurse observe in a patient whose feed rate was too high?

    A. More than five stools per day or 500 mL in 24 hours
    B. Evidence of coarse crackles auscultated throughout the lung fields
    C. Blood glucose levels greater than 180 mg/dL (10 mmol/L)
    D. Skin irritation and breakdown around the jejunostomy site

23. The patient's family asks what outcome to expect for their father who is experiencing an acute gastrointestinal bleed due to peptic ulcer disease. Which nursing statement identifies the priority for patient care?

    A. "The goal of care is to stop the bleeding, maintain a normal fluid balance, and maintain a normal hemodynamic state for your father."
    B. "Care is focused on finding the cause of your father's peptic ulcer disease and then applying preventative strategies."
    C. "It's important to understand that we may not be able to stop the bleeding and you may need to make some difficult choices for care."
    D. "I cannot speak directly to your father's care and treatment but I will ask the healthcare provider to come and see you."

24. A patient develops a physiologic stress ulcer after surgery. The nurse reviews the patient chart and notes that he was not prescribed preventative therapy prior to surgery. Which medication would the nurse look for in the patient medication record to confirm this?

    A. Ibuprofen
    B. Pantoprazole
    C. Sucralfate
    D. Misoprostol

25. The nurse is reassessing a patient admitted with a gastric ulcer for complications. What would be a clinical sign of gastric outlet obstruction?

    A. Sudden and severe abdominal pain
    B. Vomiting bright-red blood
    C. Projectile vomiting
    D. Stiff, board-like abdomen

26. A patient who is admitted to a medical unit for peptic ulcer disease completed antibiotic therapy to treat a *Helicobacter pylori* infection. What test will evaluate whether this therapy has been successful?

    A. Barium contrast study
    B. Biopsy via endoscopy
    C. Serum or whole blood antibody test
    D. Urea breath test

(See answers next page.)

22. A) More than five stools per day or 500 mL in 24 hours

Patients whose enteral feeding rate is too high will have more than three to five stools per day (or an overall total greater than 500 mL of loose stool). They may also have abdominal distension or pain. Coarse crackles in the lung fields would be evidenced in a patient experiencing fluid overload via a parental route or with a history of renal or heart failure. Hyperglycemia is not related to the rate of feeding. Increased rates of feeding are not linked to skin breakdown around the jejunostomy site.

23. A) "The goal of care is to stop the bleeding, maintain a normal fluid balance, and maintain a normal hemodynamic state for your father."

It is appropriate for the nurse to complete family teaching regarding the care of an acute gastrointestinal bleed. The focus of care is to stop the source and to maintain normovolemia and hemodynamic status. Identifying the cause of the ulcers will be integrated into the care plan, but the main priority is to stop the bleeding. Acute gastrointestinal bleeding is treatable and the family does not need to be prompted to think about palliation for this patient. It is in the scope of practice of the nurse to discuss goals for care but not the prognosis of the patient.

24. B) Pantoprazole

Prevention of physiologic stress ulcers involves the use of antisecretory agents such as proton pump inhibitors. Pantoprazole is one of the most common medications for this use. The nurse should review the patient's chart for this class of medication. Ibuprofen increases the risk of ulcers. Sucralfate would be used to help treat an existing ulcer. Misoprostol is given to patients who receive nonsteroidal anti-inflammatory drugs (NSAIDs) and may be at high risk for developing ulcers.

25. C) Projectile vomiting

Gastric outlet obstruction results from the increased contractile force needed to empty the stomach. This results in hypertrophy of the stomach and atony. The narrowing of the pylorus can result in food staying in the stomach for prolonged periods. This may cause projectile vomiting, weight loss, thirst, and bad taste in the patient's mouth from food that has been in the stomach for days. Sudden and severe abdominal pain is a sign of perforation. Vomiting bright red blood is a sign of hemorrhaging. Stiff, board-like abdomen would indicate perforation and bleeding.

26. D) Urea breath test

The urea breath test measures the presence of *H. pylori*. Barium contrast studies and endoscopic biopsy are used to detect the presence of peptic ulcers. Serum or whole blood antibody tests can be used to detect immunoglobulin G (IgG), the most prevalent antibody, but levels remain elevated in the blood after the infection has resolved.

27. A patient with peptic ulcer disease is attending an ambulatory care clinic for treatment. Which of the following statements regarding the treatment of this condition is true?

    A. It will take 2 to 3 weeks to heal the ulcer completely.

    B. The ulcer pain should decrease in 3 to 6 days with treatment.

    C. Ulcer healing is determined by the absence of *Helicobacter pylori*.

    D. The patient can resume aspirin use after treatment.

28. Which of the following are clinical signs of bile reflux gastritis that should be reported to the healthcare provider immediately?

    A. Sweating and palpitations after eating with an intense urge to defecate

    B. A significant drop in postprandial blood glucose levels

    C. Bowel incontinence

    D. Distress and intense vomiting after meals

29. Which of the following is considered an expected outcome of treatment for a patient with ulcerative colitis?

    A. The patient reports fewer and firmer stools.

    B. The patient rates their abdominal pain as 5/10 on a pain scale.

    C. The patient reports weight loss associated with dietary changes.

    D. The patient reports being able to eat half of a meal.

30. A patient is experiencing sphincter spasm after a hemorrhoidectomy. The nurse administers narcotic analgesics to treat the pain. What is an appropriate secondary nursing action?

    A. Assess for anal fissures or bruising around the surgical area.

    B. Administer an enema to prevent constipation and added pressure in the rectum.

    C. Administer a warm sitz bath for comfort and to keep the anal area clean.

    D. Encourage the patient to resist the urge to defecate until the pain subsides.

31. A patient has recurring pilonidal wounds between the skin and the buttocks. Based on the characteristics of pilonidal wounds, which factor impacts wound healing the most?

    A. Surrounding hair growing into the wound bed

    B. Amount of time the patient sits during the day

    C. Amount of pain medication needed prior to dressing changes

    D. Running or walking for long periods

32. A patient is in the icteric phase of hepatitis. The nurse would expect to evaluate:

    A. Fever and urticaria.

    B. Anorexia, nausea, and vomiting.

    C. Malaise and easy fatigability.

    D. The level of jaundice and bilirubinuria.

(See answers next page.)

27. B) The ulcer pain should decrease in 3 to 6 days with treatment.

The ulcer pain should decrease in 3 to 6 days. However, treatment should last a total of 3 to 9 weeks. Ulcer healing can be confirmed by endoscopic examination. For this patient, aspirin therapy will not be recommended in the future because of the ulcer history.

28. D) Distress and intense vomiting after meals

Gastric surgery that involves the pylorus can result in reflux alkaline gastritis. Prolonged contact with bile salts causes damage to the gastric mucosa. Patients have continuous epigastric distress and vomiting after meals. Vomiting does not relieve the symptoms. Sweating, palpitations, and an intense urge to defecate are signs of dumping syndrome. A drop in postprandial blood glucose levels indicates postprandial hypoglycemia. Bowel incontinence is not a common complication but may be associated with dumping syndrome if the patient is unable to access the bathroom in time.

29. A) The patient reports fewer and firmer stools.

Expected outcomes include the patient reporting fewer and firmer stools. Pain should be absent. The patient should be gaining weight. The patient should be able to eat a full meal.

30. C) Administer a warm sitz bath for comfort and to keep the anal area clean.

The patient should be encouraged to have a warm sitz bath to help keep the area clean and promote comfort after surgery. Assessing for fissures will not help with additional pain management. An enema would not be appropriate; oral stool softeners are prescribed instead. It is important to aid the patient's defection and not inhibit it.

31. A) Surrounding hair growing into the wound bed

A pilonidal (nest of hair) wound has several openings and is lined with epithelium and hair. The movement of the buttocks causes short wiry hair to penetrate the skin, forming a cyst or abscess that leads to an open wound. Hair growth has the greatest impact on healing and hair surrounding the wound should be clipped. The patient should limit sitting or switch to side-lying positions. These wounds are painful and analgesic will be required prior to dressing changes. Running or walking for long periods can cause rubbing or shearing of the wound.

32. D) The level of jaundice and bilirubinuria.

Hepatitis infections have three phases: preicteric, icteric, and posticteric. In the icteric phase, jaundice develops. It may also manifest with dark urine, bilirubinuria, light stools, and pruritus. Fever, urticaria, anorexia, nausea, and vomiting occur in the preicteric phase. Malaise and easy fatigability occur in the posticteric phase.

33. A family is exposed to hepatitis A at a local deli. Which statement by the parents demonstrates an understanding of the recommended treatment path for this exposure?

   A. "There is no prophylactic treatment for this condition."
   B. "We will all need to be vaccinated for hepatitis A."
   C. "There is a special drug that can be administered to give us immunity 1 to 2 weeks after exposure."
   D. "It is important for our family to be hospitalized to observe the infection."

34. The nurse is completing patient teaching regarding the treatment of *Helicobacter pylori* infection that will occur over 14 days. Which of the following patient statements demonstrates an understanding of this approach to drug therapy?

   A. "I need to take just this one antibiotic pill every day for 2 weeks."
   B. "I will take four drugs for 14 days and I need to ensure that I don't skip any days."
   C. "A proton pump inhibitor will help promote healing while I take antibiotic therapy."
   D. "If I have an allergy to penicillin, I cannot use this type of drug therapy."

35. A patient with appendicitis is awaiting surgery. Nursing interventions for this patient should include:

   A. Providing a warm compress or hot water bottle for nonpharmacologic treatment of abdominal pain.
   B. Administering a laxative prior to surgery.
   C. Assessing the patient for any signs of peritonitis.
   D. Ensuring that the patient is taking a clear fluid diet prior to surgery.

36. How should the nurse position a patient with peritonitis to help decrease their pain and discomfort?

   A. Place the patient in Fowler's position with their knees flexed.
   B. Position the patient on their left side with a pillow between their legs.
   C. Assist the patient to roll over into a prone position.
   D. Lay the patient in a supine position.

37. A patient has been prescribed sulfasalazine to treat ulcerative colitis. A critical fact to teach the patient about this drug is:

   A. Vomiting is a common occurrence in patients taking this medication.
   B. It is common to have frequent headaches when taking this medication.
   C. This medication may cause sensitivity to sunlight.
   D. This medication may cause a dangerously low white blood count.

38. A patient with diverticulitis is prescribed a low-residue diet. Which of the following meals would be appropriate for this type of diet?

   A. Greek yogurt with fruit, whole wheat toast, and orange juice with pulp
   B. Jell-O, clear broth, and tea
   C. Cream of Wheat cereal, canned pears, and a poached egg
   D. Cream of potato soup, milk, and ice cream

(See answers next page.)

33. C) "There is a special drug that can be administered to give us immunity 1 to 2 weeks after exposure."
Hepatitis A exposure is treated with immunoglobulin therapy. It provides temporary passive immunity and is effective in preventing hepatitis A if given within 1 to 2 weeks of exposure. Vaccination for hepatitis A is a preventative measure. Hospitalization only occurs if complications are present.

34. B) "I will take four drugs for 14 days and I need to ensure that I don't skip any days."
Quadruple drug therapy for *H. pylori* includes the use of a proton pump inhibitor, bismuth, tetracycline, and metronidazole for 14 days. All treatment for *H. pylori* includes multidrug therapy of three or more medications. Penicillin is not used for this bacterium.

35. C) Assessing the patient for any signs of peritonitis.
The nurse should assess for signs of peritonitis, which may be present if the appendix has ruptured or if the infection is worsening. Application of heat can cause the appendix to rupture. Laxatives or enemas increase peristalsis and can lead to perforation of the appendix. The patient should not have anything by mouth prior to surgery.

36. A) Place the patient in Fowler's position with their knees flexed.
The patient can be positioned with their knees flexed to help decrease the amount of pressure on the abdomen. A quiet, restful environment should also be promoted. The other positions may put increased force or weight on the abdomen and cause increased pain.

37. D) This medication may cause a dangerously low white blood count.
Sulfasalazine is an anti-inflammatory drug for the treatment of ulcerative colitis. It may cause agranulocytosis, a dangerously low white blood cell count, so frequent complete blood counts with a differential should be taken. This is a critical factor to note when educating the patient, because it is a life-threatening side effect. This medication also causes vomiting, frequent headaches, and sensitivity to sunlight.

38. C) Cream of Wheat cereal, canned pears, and a poached egg
A low-residue diet provides food low in fiber, which will result in a reduced amount of fecal material in the lower intestinal tract. Cream of Wheat, canned pears, and a poached egg are included in a low-residue diet. Whole-wheat toast is restricted due to its fiber content. A clear fluid diet does not provide appropriate nutrition. Cream of potato soup, milk, and icecream are considered part of a full fluid diet, which are liquid foods or foods that turn to liquid at room temperature.

39. A male patient recently had bowel surgery with the creation of a colostomy and removal of the rectum. The patient asks the nurse how this surgery will affect his sexual health. Which nursing statement outlines the physiologic links between ostomy surgery and sexual health?

    A. "Resection of the rectum can damage the parasympathetic nervous system and influence your ability to have an erection."
    B. "The ostomy surgery will not inhibit your sexual functioning, but is important to maintain a healthy body image."
    C. "The creation of the ostomy disrupts the sympathetic nervous system and will inhibit your ability to have an orgasm."
    D. "It is important to discuss your sexual health with your partners and show them your ostomy."

40. The nurse is assessing the safety of a patient with a nasogastric tube attached to low intermittent suction. Which of the following assessment findings demonstrates an urgent complication related to this equipment?

    A. The patient has a potassium level of 3.3 mEq/L (3.3 mmol/L).
    B. The patient has a distended abdomen and no bowel sounds.
    C. The patient is vomiting bright green emesis.
    D. The patient is experiencing persistent nausea.

41. A patient is admitted to the medical unit for paracentesis for ascites. Which of the following nursing interventions during the procedure will help to promote patient safety?

    A. Measure the patient's abdominal girth before and after the procedure.
    B. Ensure that the patient has a full bladder prior to the procedure.
    C. Monitor temperature every 4 hours after the procedure.
    D. Evaluate the patient for hypotension, tachycardia, and diaphoresis.

42. Which of the following nursing actions would compromise the safety of a patient with acute pancreatitis?

    A. Administering morphine for pain management
    B. Administering calcium supplements
    C. Assessing bowel sounds every 4 hours
    D. Drawing daily serum blood glucose levels

43. A patient with chronic alcoholism and cirrhosis of the liver is frequently admitted to the hospital. The patient has a rare blood type and requires frequent blood transfusions. What is the nurse's ethical responsibility when caring for this patient?

    A. The nurse should determine whether other patients in this hospital require the same blood type and prioritize administration.
    B. The nurse must ethically provide the blood transfusions unless the healthcare provider deems care to be medically futile.
    C. The nurse should consult with an ethics specialist to determine how to prevent the patient from receiving the blood.
    D. The nurse may refuse to administer blood to this patient due to their noncompliance with treatment.

(See answers next page.)

39. A) "Resection of the rectum can damage the parasympathetic nervous system and influence your ability to have an erection."

The creation of an ostomy with removal of the rectum can potentially damage the parasympathetic nervous system. In men, this leads to an inability to have an erection, so ostomy surgeries do physiologically influence sexual health and functioning. Although healthy body image is a central part of sexual health and functioning, the physiologic changes from this surgery may impact the patient the most. The sympathetic nervous system is not affected with this surgery. Although it is important to discuss sexual health issues with a partner, this question concerns the physiologic effects of an ostomy surgery on sexual function.

40. B) The patient has a distended abdomen and no bowel sounds.

The most urgent complication is the distended abdomen and absent bowel sounds. The nasogastric tube is obstructed and pressure is building up. Potassium losses are expected if the nasogastric tube is attached to suction. The nurse will need to inform the healthcare provider. Vomiting is uncommon but does happen; in these instances, the nasogastric tube is attached to suction. Patients may experience nausea if the tube is not draining or related to their underlying condition. Antiemetic therapy can be provided.

41. D) Evaluate the patient for hypotension, tachycardia, and diaphoresis.

Hypovolemia is the major risk to patient safety during a paracentesis. Hypotension, tachycardia, pallor, and diaphoresis are all signs that this is occurring. Measuring abdominal girth helps to determine how much fluid has been removed. The patient should void prior to the procedure to help avoid puncturing the bladder. Temperature should be monitored with vital signs every 15 minutes for the first 2 hours and every hour thereafter.

42. A) Administering morphine for pain management

Morphine should not be used for pain management in patients with acute pancreatitis because it can cause an increase of pressure in the sphincter of Oddi, which can worsen the condition. Patients develop hypocalcemia in this condition, so calcium supplementation is necessary. Bowel sounds should be assessed every 4 hours. Daily serum blood glucose levels should be drawn to assess damage to beta cells of the islets of Langerhans in the pancreas.

43. B) The nurse must ethically provide the blood transfusions unless the healthcare provider deems care to be medically futile.

The nurse has an ethical responsibility to provide nursing care to the patient. Alcoholism has a behavioral component, but it is still a chronic illness. A medical healthcare provider must determine that treatment is medically futile. It is not in the nurse's scope of practice to triage scarce resources. The nurse can consult with the ethics board or the healthcare provider, but the consultation should not be to prevent the patient from receiving care; rather, it should be done to examine the scarcity and use of resources.

44. A nurse has returned to work after a leave for the treatment of severe pancreatitis and is caring for a patient with the same condition. The nurse finds they are frequently sharing their own illness experience with the patient. What should the nurse do in this situation?

    A. Ask to be assigned to another patient.

    B. Speak to the nursing union in case the patient complains about the interactions.

    C. Continue to use their experience to help provide patient support.

    D. Reflect on how to better maintain professional boundaries in care.

45. The nurse caring for a patient with end-stage liver failure is delegating tasks to an unlicensed care provider. Which of the following tasks would be appropriate to delegate?

    A. Assess for signs of hematuria.

    B. Measure fluid drained during paracentesis.

    C. Collect a urine sample to measure protein levels.

    D. Ambulate the patient after the patient receives a narcotic analgesic.

46. A 35-year-old female patient admitted to hospital with upper gastrointestinal bleeding is ready for discharge home. What area of teaching should the nurse address to help prevent future bleeding episodes?

    A. Smoking and alcohol cessation, taking prescribed medications

    B. Increased antacid use with meals to prevent ulcers

    C. Regular intake of aspirin to prevent clotting

    D. Supplement nonsteroidal anti-inflammatory drug (NSAID) use with misoprostol

47. A patient with a history of liver failure and esophageal varices asks the nurse how to prevent future bleeding episodes. Which of the following health-promoting activities should the nurse recommend?

    A. Avoid the use of acetaminophen.

    B. Reduce alcohol consumption to allow the liver to heal.

    C. Treat respiratory infections promptly, because severe coughing and sneezing can cause rebleeding.

    D. Increase dietary iron intake to help raise hemoglobin and red blood cell levels.

(See answers next page.)

44. D) Reflect on how to better maintain professional boundaries in care.

The nurse needs to reflect on how to maintain better professional boundaries. It would not be necessary to be assigned to another patient. The nurse does not need to contact the nursing union, just reflect on a better use of boundaries. Using personal experience may inhibit the patient sharing details of their condition or impede therapeutic dialogue.

45. C) Collect a urine sample to measure protein levels.

The unlicensed care provider can collect a urine sample. The nurse cannot delegate assessment to the unlicensed care provider, including assessing for hematuria or measuring fluid. The unlicensed care provider cannot ambulate the patient after the patient receives a narcotic analgesic because this would also involve patient assessment.

46. A) Smoking and alcohol cessation, taking prescribed medications

A patient with one major bleeding episode is likely to have another. The patient should stop smoking, limit alcohol, decrease stress, and take her prescribed medications. Antacid use does not prevent ulcers; it promotes the healing of ulcers by decreasing the gastric pH. Aspirin is avoided because it is a gastric irritant. Misoprostol is used to help combat the effects of NSAIDs on the gastrointestinal tract, but it should not be used in women of childbearing age.

47. C) Treat respiratory infections promptly, because severe coughing and sneezing can cause rebleeding.

To prevent future bleeding episodes, it is important to treat respiratory infections right away, because severe coughing and sneezing can increase portal pressure and rupture varices. The patient would avoid acetaminophen to prevent further liver failure; the use of this medication is not directly linked to esophageal bleeding. A patient with liver failure should avoid alcohol. Increasing dietary iron may help with increasing red blood cell production, but it will not help to prevent future bleeding episodes.

Pulmonary System

1. The nurse is caring for a patient with a chest tube. What should the nurse do if the tube becomes disconnected from the drainage system?

    A. Immerse the chest tube in sterile water until the system is reestablished.
    B. Clamp the chest tube with a hemostat until the system is reestablished.
    C. Strip the chest tube and insert it into the drainage system.
    D. Elevate the drainage system above the level of the patient's chest, reconnect the chest tube, and have the patient cough.

2. An 85-year-old woman is admitted from her nursing home and is diagnosed with acute bronchitis and dehydration. Which order by the provider should the nurse question?

    A. Acetaminophen
    B. Humidifier in room
    C. Penicillin
    D. Encourage fluid intake

3. The patient arrives at the unit with a nursing diagnosis of impaired gas exchange related to fluid and exudate accumulation within the lung and surrounding lung tissue. Which blood gas values would the nurse likely find?

    A. pH 7.45, PCO_2 45 mmHg, PO_2 98 mmHg, HCO_3 26 nmol/L
    B. pH 7.45, PCO_2 43 mmHg, PO_2 96 mmHg, HCO_3 26 nmol/L
    C. pH 7.30, PCO_2 55 mmHg, PO_2 80 mmHg, HCO_3 25 nmol/L
    D. pH 7.49, PCO_2 40 mmHg, PO_2 85 mmHg, HCO_3 29 nmol/L

4. What breath sounds would be present in a patient with consolidation from pneumonia?

    A. Bronchial
    B. Bronchovesicular
    C. Vesicular
    D. No breath sounds

5. The nurse is preparing the teaching plan for a patient with active tuberculosis (TB). The patient should be instructed to:

    A. Isolate himself from the household for 2 to 3 weeks after starting medication therapy.
    B. Dispose of used tissues in plastic bags.
    C. Avoid contact with individuals outside of the household for 12 months.
    D. Take sputum cultures every 6 months.

1. A) Immerse the chest tube in sterile water until the system is reestablished.

Immersing the tube establishes a water seal, allows air to escape, and prevents air from reentering. Clamping prevents air or fluid from escaping and increases the risk of a pneumothorax. Stripping the chest tube may result in extreme negative pressure. The tube must be kept below the level of the patient's chest to promote drainage.

2. C) Penicillin

Bronchitis is often caused by a virus, rather than bacteria. Prescribing an antibiotic would not be the first choice in treatment; instead, the symptoms would be managed. To decrease any temperature, acetaminophen can be administered. Moist air delivered through a humidifier will help relieve coughing, which is usually present in bronchitis. Because the patient is dehydrated, encouraging fluid intake will assist in the rehydration process.

3. C) pH 7.30, PCO_2 55 mmHg, PO_2 80 mmHg, HCO_3 25 nmol/L

This blood gas with a pH 7.30, PCO_2 55 mmHg, PO_2 80 mmHg, and HCO_3 25 nmol/L demonstrates respiratory acidosis, which is related to poor gas exchange and retained carbon dioxide. The blood gas with a pH 7.45, PCO_2 45 mmHg, PO_2 98 mmHg, and HCO_3 26 nmol/L is within normal range. The blood gas with a pH 7.45, PCO_2 43 mmHg, PO_2 96 mmHg, and HCO_3 26 nmol/L is within normal range. The blood gas with a pH 7.49, PCO_2 40 mmHg, PO_2 85 mmHg, and HCO_3 29 nmol/L is the result of metabolic alkalosis.

4. D) No breath sounds

Consolidated areas of the lung do not have an exchange of oxygen, so there is no air flow and therefore no sounds.

5. B) Dispose of used tissues in plastic bags.

Use plastic disposal bags for dirty tissues to prevent spread of the virus. Family members have been exposed to the patient's virus before treatment and do not require isolation. After taking medications for 6 months, the patient may come in contact with the public. Sputum cultures should be done every 2 weeks.

6. Which of the following is the correct order in which to perform an assessment of the lungs and thorax?

   A. Visual inspection, auscultation, percussion, palpation
   B. Visual inspection, percussion, palpation, auscultation
   C. Visual inspection, percussion, auscultation, palpation
   D. Visual inspection, palpation, percussion, auscultation

7. A patient is experiencing impaired oxygenation and respiratory distress due to pulmonary fibrosis. How should the nurse position the patient?

   A. Place the patient in high Fowler's position.
   B. Place the patient in a prone position.
   C. Place the patient in supine position.
   D. Place the patient in semi-Fowler's position slightly turned toward the right side.

8. The nurse is planning to obtain arterial blood gases. What test should the nurse perform before collecting the sample?

   A. Echocardiogram
   B. Pulse oximetry
   C. Allen test
   D. Pulmonary function test

9. A patient presents with tachycardia, cyanosis, and chest pain. The nurse formulates a diagnosis of impaired gas exchange due to unknown cause. Which of the following tests should the nurse prepare the patient for?

   A. Pulmonary function test
   B. Pulse oximetry
   C. Bronchoscopy
   D. Ventilation/perfusion (VQ) lung scan

10. A patient with chronic obstructive pulmonary disease (COPD) has a decreased level of consciousness, labored breathing, and a respiratory rate of eight breaths/min. The patient is on oxygen via nasal prongs at 6 L/min. What is a critical nursing intervention for this patient?

    A. Call the rapid response team.
    B. Increase oxygen to 8 L/min.
    C. Obtain a full set of vital signs.
    D. Switch to an oxygen face mask.

11. A patient with pneumonia is admitted with blood gas values of pH 7.40, PCO_2 40 mmHg, PO_2 96 mmHg, and HCO_3 24 nmol/L. What should be a priority nursing diagnosis for this patient?

    A. Impaired gas exchange due to respiratory failure
    B. Impaired tissue perfusion due to pneumonia
    C. Risk of anxiety related to pneumonia
    D. At risk for impaired gas exchange related to pneumonia

(See answers next page.)

6. D) Visual inspection, palpation, percussion, auscultation

Data is collected in the order of inspection, palpation, percussion, and auscultation. Visualization may identify areas of decreased muscle movement, tachypnea, or dyspnea. Palpating the chest helps to identify specific areas for percussion. Data collected during percussion may indicate areas for specific attention during auscultation.

7. A) Place the patient in high Fowler's position.

Patients in respiratory distress should be placed in high Fowler's position. This allows for chest expansion and decreased work of breathing. Prone position is only used in patients in advanced respiratory failure who may be experiencing acute respiratory distress syndrome (ARDS). These patients are typically mechanically ventilated. Supine position would not help to relieve distress and will not improve oxygenation. Turning the patient on the right side may cause further distress and oxygen impairment.

8. C) Allen test

The Allen test is used to determine whether there is adequate collateral circulation in the hand before drawing blood. An echocardiogram is used to assess heart movement, and pulse oximetry is used to assess arterial blood oxygenation. A pulmonary function test is used to differentiate between obstructive and restrictive lung disease.

9. D) Ventilation/perfusion (VQ) lung scan

A VQ lung scan will detect the presence of a pulmonary embolism. The patient is demonstrating symptoms consistent with this condition. A pulmonary function test shows whether the patient has restrictive or obstructive pulmonary disease. Pulse oximetry is used to assess arterial blood oxygenation and indicates how stable the patient is. A bronchoscopy would be used to visualize or biopsy the main bronchus, not the pulmonary system. An echocardiogram is used to assess heart movement and may show tachycardia or a dysrhythmia (but will not diagnose the condition).

10. A) Call the rapid response team.

Some patients with COPD will experience CO_2 retention (due to chronically high levels of CO_2 in the body). In this case, they depend on lack of O_2 rather than increased CO_2 in the body to stimulate their respiratory drive. Too much oxygen will decrease the hypoxic drive and lead to respiratory depression. The rapid response team should be called to help manage the situation. Increasing the oxygen to 8 L/min and utilizing an oxygen face mask would further decrease the hypoxic drive and lead to worsening respiratory depression. The nurse should obtain a full set of vital signs after activating the rapid response team.

11. D) At risk for impaired gas exchange related to pneumonia

This is a normal blood gas, so there is no need to change the patient care focus. This patient is at risk for impaired gas exchange due to pneumonia and needs to be monitored. This patient is not demonstrating signs of respiratory failure in the blood gas or evidence of impaired tissue perfusion. Although there is a chance there may be a risk for anxiety related to pneumonia, impaired gas exchange is a primary diagnosis.

12. After a flight from Europe, a patient is admitted to the floor with breathlessness, pleuritic pain, apprehension, a slight fever, and productive cough with blood-streaked sputum. Nursing care includes which of the following interventions?

    A. Administer vitamin K.
    B. Apply sequential compression device.
    C. Maintain bed rest.
    D. Prepare for immediate intubation.

13. The nurse is caring for a patient with persistent inflammation and narrowing of the nasal mucosa. Which of the following patient actions would impede the ability to heal from this condition?

    A. Avoiding exposure to smoke in the environment
    B. Taking dimenhydrinate to treat symptoms
    C. Irrigating the nasal passages with 5 mL of salt water
    D. Drinking six to eight glasses of water per day

14. A patient has a 30-year habit of smoking a pack of cigarettes per day. Which of the following blood gases would the nurse expect on assessment?

    A. Respiratory acidosis
    B. Respiratory alkalosis
    C. Metabolic acidosis
    D. Metabolic alkalosis

15. A patient who is having an acute asthmatic attack is not responding to their regular rescue medication. The patient's oxygen saturation is 68% on 10 L/min of oxygen and has noted wheezing and stridor. Which of the following medications should the nurse expect the healthcare provider to order?

    A. Albuterol administered via nebulizer
    B. Theophylline intravenous (IV) infusion
    C. Ipratropium administered via metered dose inhaler
    D. Salmeterol administered via nebulizer

16. A patient develops acute respiratory failure related to Guillain–Barré syndrome. The nurse identifies that the patient is at risk for ineffective airway clearance. What intervention should the nurse implement?

    A. Reposition the patient every 2 hours.
    B. Elevate the foot of the bed.
    C. Obtain an order for heparin.
    D. Provide sedation.

17. A patient with hypopnea caused by an opioid overdose presents with an acid–base alteration. The nurse expects that the patient will exhibit which scenario?

    A. Hyperventilation with respiratory acidosis
    B. Hypoventilation with respiratory acidosis
    C. Hypoventilation with respiratory alkalosis
    D. Respiratory acidosis with normal oxygen levels

(See answers next page.)

12. B) Apply sequential compression device.

The goal is to prevent further development of emboli. A compression device assists in the prevention of venous stasis. Vitamin K would counteract thrombolytic therapy. Ambulation, not bed rest, is encouraged to prevent venous stasis. No data is presented that supports the need for intubation.

13. B) Taking dimenhydrinate to treat symptoms

Classic (first-generation) antihistamines can worsen symptoms of sinusitis. Patients should be taught to avoid smoke, irrigate the nasal passages with salt water or steam inhalations, and increase their daily fluid intake to at least 6 to 8 glasses of water daily.

14. A) Respiratory acidosis

Respiratory acidosis is seen in patients with emphysema due to retention of carbon dioxide in the body from air trapped in the alveoli. This increases carbonic acid and results in a decreased or acidotic pH level. Respiratory alkalosis is commonly observed in patients with hyperventilation or pneumonia. Metabolic acidosis can be linked to kidney disease or an acute poisoning. Metabolic alkalosis is linked to repeated vomiting and severe dehydration.

15. B) Theophylline intravenous (IV) infusion

Rescue medications for asthma include rapid beta 2 agonist medications. The most common is albuterol. If a patient is not responding to this therapy and is clinically declining, another potent bronchodilation medication may be used. Theophylline is a methylxanthine and results in potent bronchodilation. It is only used for patients with refractory asthma. Ipratropium is an anticholinergic drug and may be used with a beta 2 agonist. However, its mechanism of action is not strong enough in this type of clinical decline. Salmeterol is a long-term beta 2 agonist and will help with maintenance and management.

16. A) Reposition the patient every 2 hours.

Repositioning the patient will facilitate mobilization of secretions. Elevating the foot of the bed would not be beneficial. Venous thromboembolism prophylaxis is ordered to prevent complications of immobility. Sedation is an intervention to manage anxiety, and administration of sedatives increases the risk for retained secretions.

17. B) Hypoventilation with respiratory acidosis

Hypoventilation impairs elimination of carbon dioxide, so respiratory acidosis occurs. Opioid sedation results in hypoventilation, not hyperventilation. *Hypoxemia* refers to a reduction of PO_2 in the arterial blood from depressed respirations or hypoventilation.

18. A patient demonstrates a partial arterial oxygen level (PO_2) of 55 mmHg while on a fraction of inspired oxygen (FiO_2) of 0.8. The patient is on 15 L of oxygen via nonrebreather mask. What is a priority nursing intervention?

    A. Call the healthcare provider immediately and prepare for endotracheal intubation.
    B. Call the respiratory therapist.
    C. Request an x-ray of the patient's chest.
    D. Assist the patient to lie in a prone position.

19. The nurse is providing preoperative teaching to a patient on postoperative breathing exercises. Which immediate postoperative respiratory disorder is the nurse attempting to prevent?

    A. Pneumothorax
    B. Pneumonia
    C. Bronchitis
    D. Atelectasis

20. The nurse includes teaching which of the following interventions for a patient with emphysema?

    A. Use an orthopneic position with the bed in a low Fowler's position.
    B. Use pursed-lip and diaphragmatic breathing.
    C. Use coordinated breathing by inhaling through the mouth and exhaling through the nose.
    D. Use 6 L of humidified oxygen via nasal cannula.

21. A patient infected with *Mycobacterium tuberculosis* expresses concern regarding the care of an elderly relative after discharge. What should the nurse tell the patient as part of discharge planning related to the care of an elderly relative?

    A. "You can perform all activities when you go home that you did before your hospitalization."
    B. "It is likely that your family members are already infected, so isolation is not required."
    C. "If you are concerned about your ability to care for your relative, I will consult social services for assistance."
    D. "You have no worries; the medication will cure the tuberculosis."

22. A patient is diagnosed with sarcoidosis and admitted to the medical–surgical floor. Which order from the provider requires additional investigation by the nurse?

    A. Culture new skin lesions
    B. Place tuberculin skin test (purified protein derivative [PPD])
    C. Administer oral vitamin D
    D. Check visual acuity

(*See answers next page.*)

18. A) Call the healthcare provider immediately and prepare for endotracheal intubation.

The nurse would calculate a PF ratio (PO_2 divided by FiO_2) to determine the oxygenation at a cellular level. This patient has a PF ratio of 69. This is indicative of acute lung injury and potentially acute respiratory distress syndrome. The healthcare provider should be called because directives for potential intubation may be needed. A respiratory therapist can be consulted after the healthcare provider is made aware of the situation and has made treatment recommendations. A chest x-ray will be performed after intubation as it is not a priority action. Changing the patient's position will not help increase the PO_2 levels. The patient requires advanced intervention.

19. D) Atelectasis

Atelectasis refers to an incomplete expansion of a lung or portion of a lung, which in rare cases can occur after intubation. Lung expansion is limited by a patient's splinting due to pain. Pneumothorax is the presence of air in the pleural space. Pneumonia is the inflammation of the parenchymal structure of the lung. Bronchitis is the obstruction of the airways from hypersecretions of mucus.

20. B) Use pursed-lip and diaphragmatic breathing.

Pursed-lip breathing enhances airflow and helps to prevent airway collapse. High levels of oxygen will decrease the ventilatory drive. *Coordinated breathing* refers to inhaling through the nose and exhaling through the mouth. The low Fowler's position does not work with an orthopneic position.

21. C) "If you are concerned about your ability to care for your relative, I will consult social services for assistance."

Discharge planning encompasses the patient's postacute care and the significant factors that affect transition from the hospital. Activities should be gradually increased. The family has been exposed, but the nurse should not suggest that they are absolutely infected. The last comment negates the patient's concerns.

22. A) Culture new skin lesions

Sarcoidosis can result in lesions that appear outside of the lungs. Lesions may be found on the eyes and skin. Skin lesions should be biopsied to determine whether they are sarcoidosis lesions; however, a skin culture would not provide this information. Visual acuity should be checked to assess for signs of eye involvement. In addition, all patients with sarcoidosis should be tested for tuberculosis. Vitamin D and calcium are often prescribed due to associated deficits.

23. A patient is admitted with ipsilateral chest pain, increased respiratory rate, dyspnea, and accumulation of air in the chest cavity. The nurse prepares the patient for treatment for which of the following respiratory disorders?

    A. Pneumothorax
    B. Atelectasis
    C. Acute asthma
    D. Empyema

24. The nurse is suctioning a mechanically ventilated patient via an endotracheal tube when the patient becomes bradycardic. What is a priority nursing intervention?

    A. Continue suctioning the patient for another 10 seconds.
    B. Withdraw the catheter and hyperoxygenate the patient.
    C. Call the rapid response team.
    D. Monitor the patient for increasing respiratory distress.

25. A nurse is caring for a patient with chronic obstructive pulmonary disease (COPD) who has impaired gas exchange related to air trapping in the alveoli. The patient has an oxygen saturation of 66% on room air and is breathing through the mouth. Which oxygen system should be used to support the patient based on this nursing diagnosis?

    A. Face tent
    B. Nasal cannula with humidity
    C. Venturi mask
    D. Simple mask

26. What symptoms are associated with tuberculosis?

    A. Weight gain, night sweats, fever, cough
    B. Chest and lower back pain
    C. Chills, low-grade fever, night sweats, cough with blood
    D. Chills, high temperatures, night sweats, cough with blood

27. A patient is admitted with symptoms of sudden onset of fever, cough, weakness, and myalgias. The patient's nursing diagnosis is potential for ineffective breathing pattern related to complex factors. The nurse instructs the patient to follow which activity?

    A. Drink very hot tea.
    B. Rest quietly.
    C. Limit fluid intake.
    D. Take a hot bath.

28. A patient with an accumulation of viscid mucus in the bronchi is admitted to the floor. The nurse assesses the patient to have ineffective airway clearance related to thick mucus secondary to cystic fibrosis. The nurse would instruct the patient on the use of which device?

    A. Peak flow meter
    B. Incentive spirometer
    C. Bilevel positive airway pressure (BiPap)
    D. Flutter valve

(See answers next page.)

23. A) Pneumothorax

Pneumothorax is the presence of air in the pleural space with symptoms of ipsilateral chest pain, increased heart rate, dyspnea, and presence of air. *Atelectasis* is the incomplete expansion of the lung, which results in wheezing, coughing, and shallow breathing. Acute asthma is generalized throughout the entire lung with a distressed breathing pattern of shortness of breath. Empyema is the accumulation of pus in the pleural space resulting in painful breathing, fever, and a dry cough.

24. B) Withdraw the catheter and hyperoxygenate the patient.

Bradycardia during endotracheal suctioning is a sign of a vasovagal response. The correct way to suction is to suction for up to 10 seconds. The patient has exhibited respiratory distress. If the rate continues to drop, the rapid response team would be called. After treating with oxygen, the patient's status should be continuously monitored.

25. C) Venturi mask

A Venturi mask is used to deliver a precise percentage of controlled oxygen to a patient with COPD. It will also support a patient breathing through the mouth. A face tent delivery of oxygen varies based on the amount of environmental loss. A nasal cannula delivery of oxygen is dependent on the patient's breathing pattern and is not appropriate for this patient's low oxygen saturation. A simple mask will not support the level of oxygen delivery required for this patient.

26. C) Chills, low-grade fever, night sweats, cough with blood

The usual symptoms for tuberculosis include chills with low-grade temperatures, chest pain related to coughing episodes, and weight loss. Back pain and high temperatures are not normally seen in tuberculosis.

27. B) Rest quietly.

Rest decreases the oxygen requirements and reduces the rate and chance of spreading the virus from the upper to the lower respiratory tract. Drinking very hot or cold fluids may cause coughing spells, creating dyspnea and bronchospasms. Caffeine reduces the effects of some bronchodilators. Drinking large amounts of fluid helps to ensure that the function of the epithelial lining of the respiratory tract is not further compromised by dehydration; therefore, fluid intake should not be limited. Hot water increases body temperature, whereas a tepid bath helps to prevent chilling, which may aggravate and increase temperature.

28. D) Flutter valve

A flutter valve is a handheld mucus-clearance device. A peak flow meter is used to measure how air flows from the lungs in one fast blast. An incentive spirometer is used to keep lungs healthy after surgery or respiratory illness, such as pneumonia, by facilitating large, slow breaths to keep lungs expanded. BiPap is used to deliver pressurized air through a mask to regulate the breathing pattern.

29. A patient is admitted with a diagnosis of pleural effusion. How will the nurse best position the patient for a thoracentesis?

   A. Supine position with both arms extended
   B. Lying at the edge of the bed, affected side down, with the same-side arm over the head and bed elevated 45 degrees
   C. Lying at the edge of the bed, unaffected side down, with the same-side arm over the head and bed elevated 45 degrees
   D. Forward side lying position with arms and head flat

30. A patient is admitted with a history of chronic obstructive pulmonary disease. The nurse's priority for care is which of the following symptoms?

   A. Low-grade fever and cough
   B. Irritating cough and watery sputum
   C. Restlessness and confusion
   D. Nausea and vomiting

31. A family that recently returned from vacation was notified that they had been exposed to tuberculosis (TB) about 8 weeks ago. To screen for the presence of the infection, the nurse will conduct which of the following tests?

   A. Sputum culture
   B. Chest x-ray
   C. Blood culture
   D. Purified protein derivative (PPD) intradermal test

32. A nurse is caring for a patient with Legionnaires' disease. The nurse identifies which of the following as a priority of care for this patient?

   A. Dry mucous membranes in the mouth
   B. A decrease in respiratory rate from 34 to 24 breaths/min
   C. Decrease in chest wall expansion
   D. Pleuritic pain on inspiration

33. A patient on mechanical ventilation with a tracheostomy needs suctioning. The nurse performs which of the following to avoid hypoxia?

   A. Hyperoxygenate with 100% oxygen for 1 to 2 minutes before and after each suction pass.
   B. Complete suction pass in 30 seconds with pressure of 150 mmHg.
   C. Insert a fenestrated catheter with a whistle tip without suction.
   D. Limit suction pass to 60 seconds while slowly rotating the lubricated catheter.

(*See answers next page.*)

29. B) Lying at the edge of the bed, affected side down, with the same-side arm over the head and bed elevated 45 degrees

Lying at the edge of the bed with the affected side down facilitates removal of pleural fluid by widening the intercostal spaces on the affected side. Supine and flat positions are best done with ultrasound or CT guidance. Raising the arm overhead facilitates an opening space for needle insertion and narrows the space on opposite side.

30. C) Restlessness and confusion

Respiratory failure includes the following symptoms: excessive somnolence, aggressiveness, confusion, central cyanosis, and shortness of breath. Restlessness and confusion may occur early as oxygenation decreases. An irritating cough, fever, nausea, and vomiting may not be initial symptoms with respiratory failure.

31. D) Purified protein derivative (PPD) intradermal test

The administration of the PPD intradermal test determines the presence of the *Mycobacterium tuberculosis* infection organism after an initial infection after 3 to 6 weeks. Sputum cultures and chest x-rays are used to identify latent TB infection or a progression to TB disease. The blood test for TB, interferon gamma release assay, is not a blood culture.

32. C) Decrease in chest wall expansion

Legionnaires' disease is an acute bacterial pneumonia. All of these findings have the potential to be serious. Chest wall expansion reflects a possible decrease in the depth and effort of respirations, which may indicate the need for ventilation and is therefore the most urgent symptom requiring attention. Dry mucous membranes indicate dehydration. A drop in oxygen may lead to restlessness and may indicate hypoxemia. Pleuritic pain is expected with infections.

33. A) Hyperoxygenate with 100% oxygen for 1 to 2 minutes before and after each suction pass.

Administer supplemental oxygen 100% before starting and between suctioning passes to prevent hypoxemia. Suctioning events should last approximately 10 to 15 seconds, not 30 or 60 seconds. Tracheostomy tubes are fenestrated, not suction catheters.

34. The patient presents with a chronic productive cough, dyspnea, and wheezing. The nurse's assessment reveals that the patient has cyanosis, distended neck veins, and prominent epigastric pulsation. The nurse identifies that the assessment is symptomatic of which disease?

    A. Chronic bronchitis
    B. Emphysema
    C. Pneumonia
    D. Cor pulmonale

35. A patient is being admitted with pneumonia caused by methicillin-resistant *Staphylococcus aureus* (MRSA). Which is the most appropriate isolation type the nurse should implement for this patient?

    A. Reverse isolation
    B. Contact isolation
    C. Respiratory isolation
    D. Standard isolation

36. A patient is admitted to an isolation room after a diagnosis of tuberculosis. The nurse's teaching plan includes information on the most common means of transmission of the tubercle bacillus, which is which of the following?

    A. Coughing
    B. Eating utensils
    C. Milk products
    D. Hands

37. A nurse is establishing and maintaining an airway for a patient who experienced a near-drowning episode in the ocean. The nurse must recognize which of the following as a potential danger for the patient?

    A. Pulmonary edema
    B. Alkalosis
    C. Renal failure
    D. Hypovolemia

38. A nurse provides teaching to a patient newly diagnosed with chronic obstructive pulmonary disease (COPD). Which of the following statements from the patient demonstrates an understanding of the nurse's teaching?

    A. "If I stop smoking, I can cure my condition."
    B. "I'm at risk for anemia due to hypoxia and may require blood transfusions during acute illnesses."
    C. "If I can't breathe well, I can just turn up my oxygen."
    D. "I will stop my high-intensity workout routine."

(*See answers next page.*)

34. D) Cor pulmonale
Symptoms of cor pulmonale include cyanosis, clubbing, distended neck veins, right ventricular heave or gallop, and epigastric pulsations. Symptoms of chronic bronchitis include dry cough, fatigue or malaise, postnasal drip, chest pressure, headaches, shortness of breath, and sleeping difficulty. Symptoms of emphysema include frequent lung infections, copious amounts of mucus, reduced appetite and weight loss, fatigue, cyanosis, anxiety and depression, and difficulty sleeping.

35. B) Contact isolation
Contact isolation involves the use of barrier protection (gloves, mask, gown, or protective eyewear as appropriate) whenever direct contact with any body fluid is expected. Contact precautions with good handwashing techniques are the best defense against the spread of MRSA. Reverse isolation is used to protect the patient from germs carried by staff and visitors. Respiratory isolation protects the provider from airborne droplets. Standard isolation includes gloves, masks, protective equipment, and handwashing, and is considered universal protection.

36. A) Coughing
The common means of tuberculosis transmission is droplet nuclei. The tubercle bacillus is not typically transmitted by utensils, milk products, or hands.

37. A) Pulmonary edema
Pulmonary edema may occur because of the high osmotic pressure of the aspirated ocean water. Hypoxia and acidosis (not alkalosis) may occur after a near drowning. Renal failure is not a sequela of near drowning. Hypervolemia (not hypovolemia) occurs because of the fluid drawn into the lungs by the hypertonic salt water.

38. D) "I will stop my high-intensity workout routine."
COPD may lead to pulmonary hypertension, cor pulmonale, or right ventricular heart failure. The damage has been done to the respiratory system and cannot be cured, but the elimination of smoking as an irritant is good. Phlebotomy is used to reduce blood volume if hematocrit is more than 60%. COPD patients are accustomed to an elevated level of residual carbon dioxide and do not respond to high CO_2 concentrations as the normal respiratory stimulant, instead depending on low oxygen levels to stimulate breathing. Gentle exercise, including walking, is not contraindicated in COPD patients.

39. The nurse is providing instruction on diaphragmatic breathing to a patient with chronic obstructive pulmonary disease (COPD). The nurse explains to the patient that this type of breathing will do what?

    A. Increase the breathing rate to prevent hypoxemia.
    B. Decrease the use of abdominal muscles.
    C. Encourage the use of accessory muscles to facilitate breathing.
    D. Strengthen the diaphragm.

40. The nurse auscultates the chest of a patient with a right-sided pneumothorax. What would the nurse expect to find on the assessment?

    A. Absence of breath sounds in the right thorax
    B. Bilateral inspiratory and expiratory crackles
    C. Inspiratory wheezes in the right thorax
    D. Bilateral pleural friction rub

41. As part of discharge teaching, the nurse recommends that the patient with asthma should receive the vaccines for pneumonia and flu for which of the following reasons?

    A. The vaccines produce bronchodilation and improve oxygenation.
    B. All patients are recommended to have these vaccinations.
    C. The vaccines help reduce the tachypnea in patients.
    D. Respiratory infections can cause severe hypoxia and possibly death in asthma patients.

42. A patient becomes drowsy and presents with an increase in pulse and respirations after a spontaneous pneumothorax. With a nursing diagnosis of ineffective gas exchange related to complex factors, the nurse anticipates all of the following EXCEPT:

    A. A high PO_2.
    B. Respiratory acidosis.
    C. Hypercapnia.
    D. Shortness of breath.

43. A patient has recently had chest tubes inserted. The nurse should monitor the patient for the complication of subcutaneous emphysema by performing which of the following?

    A. Compare the length of inspiration with the length of expiration.
    B. Assess for the presence of a barrel-shaped chest.
    C. Auscultate the breath sounds for crackles and rhonchi.
    D. Palpate around the chest tube insertion sites for crepitus.

(See answers next page.)

39. D) Strengthen the diaphragm

Diaphragmatic breathing focuses on using the diaphragm instead of the accessory muscles to achieve maximum inhalation and slow the respiratory rate, thereby strengthening the diaphragm.

40. A) Absence of breath sounds in the right thorax

Pneumothorax is the collapse of a lung resulting from a disruption of the negative pressure that normally exists within the space, so there is no gas exchange. No breath sounds, crackles, or wheezing are heard in the right thorax. No bilateral pleural friction rub exists because of the compression of the right lung.

41. D) Respiratory infections can cause severe hypoxia and possibly death in asthma patients.

The Centers for Disease Control and Prevention (CDC) recommends that individuals with chronic pulmonary disease, including asthma, receive these vaccines to limit influenza-related mortality and decrease transmission of the virus. Influenza and other respiratory viruses are risk factors for more severe and more frequent lower respiratory tract infections, as well as complications such as bronchiolitis, sepsis, and secondary bacterial infection.

42. A) A high PO_2.

A decreased surface area for gaseous exchange results from a pneumothorax. Carbon dioxide builds up in the blood, with the PO_2 decreasing because of the decreased surface for gas exchange. The unaffected pleural regions are not able to compensate, thus building up carbon dioxide in the blood (hypercapnia). Acidosis occurs because of the elevated PCO_2, and the patient experiences shortness of breath in an effort to obtain more air.

43. D) Palpate around the chest tube insertion sites for crepitus.

Subcutaneous emphysema occurs when air leaks from the intrapleural space through the thoracotomy or around the chest tubes into the soft tissue. Crepitus is the crackling sound heard when tissues containing gas are palpated. This is related to respiratory emphysema patterns, not subcutaneous emphysema. A barrel-shaped chest is associated with chronic obstructive pulmonary disease (COPD) due to prolonged trapping of air in the alveoli, as with emphysema. Not needed to determine crepitus, crackling and rhonchi are auscultated within the lung.

44. The nurse notes deterioration of the blood gases of a patient with chronic obstructive pulmonary disease (COPD), and respiratory failure is pending. The nurse should first assess the patient for which of the following?

    A. Bradycardia
    B. Cyanosis
    C. Mental confusion
    D. Distended neck veins

45. A patient is being prepared for a pulmonary function test. In order to determine whether the patient will breathe normally, the nurse asks the respiratory therapist to measure which of the following?

    A. Tidal volume
    B. Vital capacity
    C. Expiratory reserve
    D. Inspiratory reserve

(See answers next page.)

44. C) Mental confusion

Decreased oxygen to the vital centers in the brain results in restlessness and confusion. Tachycardia (not bradycardia) would occur as a compensatory mechanism to increase oxygen to body cells. Cyanosis is a late sign of respiratory failure. Distended veins occur with fluid volume excess and pulmonary edema.

45. A) Tidal volume

Tidal volume is the amount of air inhaled and exhaled while breathing normally. Vital capacity is the amount of air that can be forcibly expired after a deep inspiration. Expiratory reserve is the maximum amount of air that can be expired after expiration of the tidal volume. Inspiratory reserve is the maximum amount of air that can be inspired following the inspiration of the tidal volume.

Cardiovascular System

1. The nurse is providing discharge teaching to a patient who smokes and has a diagnosis of peripheral vascular disease. The nurse's teaching will include which of the following about nicotine?

   A. It constricts the peripheral vessels and increases the force of the flow.
   B. It dilates the superficial vessels and increases the force of the flow.
   C. It dilates the peripheral vessels, causing reflex constriction of visceral vessels.
   D. It constricts the superficial vessels, dilating the deep vessels.

2. The nurse should observe a patient who has undergone an endarterectomy for which of the following changes?

   A. Skin color
   B. Tissue turgor
   C. Appetite
   D. Bowel habits

3. A patient develops a thrombophlebitis while recovering from abdominal surgery. The nurse's assessment reveals this complication because of which symptom?

   A. Localized warmth and tenderness of the leg
   B. Severe pain upon extension of an extremity
   C. Pitting edema of the lower extremities
   D. Intermittent claudication

4. The nurse is going to help alleviate the distress of a patient with heart failure and pulmonary edema. What activity should the nurse assist the patient with?

   A. Encourage frequent coughing.
   B. Elevate the lower extremities.
   C. Prepare for modified postural drainage.
   D. Place the patient in an orthopneic position.

5. A patient is admitted to the hospital with a diagnosis of possible myocardial infarction. The nurse would check which of the following lab tests to find the first enzyme change for the myocardial infarction?

   A. Troponin T
   B. Total lactate dehydrogenase (LDH)
   C. Aspartate aminotransferase (AST)
   D. Alanine transaminase (ALT)

1. A) It constricts the peripheral vessels and increases the force of the flow.
Nicotine constricts the peripheral blood vessels, and the resulting increase in blood pressure impairs circulation and limits the amount of oxygen being delivered to body cells, especially in the extremities. Nicotine constricts rather than dilates the peripheral vessels. Nicotine constricts all peripheral vessels. Its primary action is vasoconstriction; it does not dilate deep vessels.

2. A) Skin color
The nurse should monitor for adequate circulation by observing skin color, pulses, and skin temperature after the removal of an arterial obstruction by an endarterectomy. Tissue turgor will be affected by alterations in hydration. Appetite is not affected by the surgery, nor are bowel habits.

3. A) Localized warmth and tenderness of the leg
The nurse's assessment for thrombophlebitis includes pain on dorsiflexion of the foot, redness, warmth, tenderness, and edema. Pain on extension of the foot is Homan's sign. Pitting edema does not occur with thrombophlebitis. Intermittent claudication may result from ischemia or peripheral vascular disease.

4. D) Place the patient in an orthopneic position.
The nurse should place the patient in an orthopneic position for maximum lung expansion because gravity reduces the pressure of the abdominal viscera on the diaphragm and lungs. Excessive coughing and mucus production are the result of the pulmonary edema and do not have to be encouraged by the nurse. Elevation of extremities should be avoided because it increases venous return, placing additional stress on the heart. Positioning for postural draining also increases venous return to the heart and does not relieve acute dyspnea.

5. A) Troponin T
The nurse would first check the troponin T because of the high specificity for myocardial cell injury; it elevates more rapidly than other enzymes. Total LDH elevates 24 to 48 hours after myocardial infarction. AST elevates 8 hours after myocardial infarction. ALT is found primarily in the liver and is used to diagnose and monitor the liver, not the heart.

6. A patient is admitted to the hospital with a diagnosis of cardiomyopathy. Upon standing, the patient's blood pressure has decreased from 165/108 mmHg to 104/60 mmHg, with the heart rate rising from 72 beats/min to 110 beats/min. The nurse instructs the patient to perform which of the following care strategies?

   A. Wear support hose continuously.
   B. Lie down for 30 minutes after taking medication.
   C. Avoid tasks that require high energy expenditures.
   D. Sit on the edge of the bed for a short time before rising.

7. The nurse walks into the patient's room and finds the patient unconscious and unresponsive. What is the first action the nurse should take?

   A. Initiate a code.
   B. Check for a radial pulse.
   C. Give four full breaths for lung inflation.
   D. Compress the lower sternum 1 minute.

8. The patient is waiting to have a repair of an abdominal aortic aneurysm. Which of the following symptoms would the nurse report immediately to the physician?

   A. Severe back pain
   B. Swelling of the arms and face
   C. High blood pressure
   D. Increased agitation

9. A nurse is caring for a patient 30 minutes after a left-heart catheterization when the patient's blood pressure begins to drop. Which potential complication does the nurse assess for?

   A. Absent distal pulses
   B. Increased pain at puncture site
   C. Nausea
   D. Bleeding or hematoma at the puncture site

10. The nurse is preparing discharge teaching for a patient with arterial insufficiency and Raynaud's disease. The nurse's teaching includes which of the following instructions?

    A. The patient should walk several times a day as part of an exercise program.
    B. The patient should keep the heat up so the environment is warm.
    C. The patient should wear thromboembolic-deterrent hose during the day.
    D. The patient should use hydrotherapy to increase oxygenation.

11. A patient is admitted to the hospital with a diagnosis of left-sided congestive heart failure (CHF). The nurse's assessment will include which of the following symptoms?

    A. Crushing chest pain
    B. Extensive peripheral edema
    C. Jugular vein distension
    D. Dyspnea on exertion

(See answers next page.)

6. D) Sit on the edge of the bed for a short time before rising.

Postural hypotension is a decrease in systolic blood pressure of more than 15% and is usually accompanied by dizziness indicating volume depletion, inadequate vasoconstriction mechanisms, and autonomic insufficiency. Sitting on the side of the bed before getting up gives the body a chance to adjust to the effects of gravity on the circulation in the upright position. Support hose would not be worn continuously and would not prevent hypotension. Lying down after taking medication would not prevent episodes of orthostatic hypotension. Energetic tasks do not prevent hypotension.

7. A) Initiate a code.

The nurse initiates the code by obtaining help immediately because the patient is unresponsive and likely will need support, potentially including cardiac and pulmonary support. The radial pulse is not used to check for a pulse. Cardiac compressions should be started before giving breaths, and two breaths should be given rather than four. Compression of the lower sternum for 1 minute is not indicated.

8. A) Severe back pain

The primary symptom of a dissecting aneurysm is a sudden, severe pain. Abdominal dissections commonly cause back pain. Many abdominal aortic aneurysms have an undetected swelling of a portion of the aorta, not the face or extremities. The patient experiencing a potential dissection would exhibit low blood pressure, not high blood pressure, and would potentially show signs of increasing loss of consciousness, due to potential blood loss upon rupture.

9. D) Bleeding or hematoma at the puncture site

The nurse understands that the loss of circulating volume from the puncture site or into the surrounding area can result in a decrease of blood pressure. Absent distal pulses indicate a blockage in an artery but are not necessarily connected to a decreased blood pressure. Pain at the puncture site is likely to stimulate increased blood pressure. Nausea is more likely to increase blood pressure.

10. B) The patient should keep the heat up so the environment is warm.

The nurse includes instructions on keeping the environment warm to prevent vasoconstriction. Wearing gloves, warm clothing, and socks would also be useful in preventing vasoconstriction. The thromboembolic-deterrent hose would not be therapeutic because of the constricting characteristics of the stockings. Excessive walking would most likely increase pain.

11. D) Dyspnea on exertion

The nurse's assessment would include a notation of dyspnea on exertion. Pulmonary congestion and edema occur because of fluid extravasation from the pulmonary capillary bed, resulting in difficulty breathing. Left-sided heart failure creates a backward effect on the pulmonary system, which leads to pulmonary congestion. Crushing chest pain is not a symptom. Peripheral edema is a symptom of right-sided heart failure, as is jugular vein distention.

12. The nurse is caring for a patient who completed a cardiac catheterization. Which of the following is a priority for nursing care?

    A. Check pulse distal to the insertion site.
    B. Check the EKG every 30 minutes.
    C. Administer oxygen.
    D. Provide for extra rest.

13. The nurse is conducting an assessment on a newly admitted patient who reports occipital headaches, blurred vision, fatigue, and increasing edema. The nurse suspects that the symptoms are related to which of the following conditions?

    A. Hypertension
    B. Hypovolemic shock
    C. Ventricular tachycardia
    D. Hypotension

14. A patient is admitted with myocarditis and asks about the prognosis of the disease. The nurse answers with which of the following responses?

    A. "A heart transplant is a very promising therapy."
    B. "A person in your situation will have good outcomes with a heart transplant. You have nothing to worry about."
    C. "The coronary artery angioplasty requires 1 to 3 days in the hospital, but there is a good outcome after the surgery."
    D. "Recovery usually happens without any special treatment."

15. A patient complains of increasing anginal pain after activity. The nurse explains to the patient that angina pectoris is a sign of which of the following?

    A. Coronary thrombosis
    B. Mitral insufficiency
    C. Myocardial ischemia
    D. Myocardial infarction

16. A patient hears the term *tachycardia* and asks what it means. The nurse describes it with which of the following terms?

    A. Irregular heartbeat
    B. Shortness of breath
    C. Fast heart rate
    D. Elevated blood pressure

17. The nurse is taking the patient's apical pulse. Where would the nurse place the stethoscope to listen?

    A. Just to the left of the median point of the sternum
    B. Between the third and fourth ribs and to the left of the sternum
    C. In the fifth intercostal space at the left midclavicular line
    D. Between the sixth and seventh ribs at the left midaxillary line

(See answers next page.)

12. A) Check pulse distal to the insertion site.

The nurse should check the pulse because the trauma at the insertion site may interfere with blood flow at the distal site. It is not necessary to check the EKG every 30 minutes after the procedure. Providing oxygen therapy is planned on an individual basis; it is not routine. Typically, no extra rest is required after the initial period of immobilization.

13. A) Hypertension

Clinical manifestations of hypertension include blurred vision, fatigue, occipital headaches, and increased edema. Hypovolemic shock presents with a rapid heartbeat, confusion, and rapid, shallow breathing. Symptoms of ventricular tachycardia include palpitations, fatigue, and chest pressure. Hypotension symptoms may include lightheadedness rather than headaches, and fatigue.

14. D) "Recovery usually happens without any special treatment."

Recovery from myocarditis is usually unremarkable. A heart transplant is not needed unless the patient is in a very late stage of the disease process. Coronary artery angioplasty with angina is indicated in patients with two-vessel disease.

15. C) Myocardial ischemia

Angina pectoris is pain in the chest that is caused by myocardial ischemia, or hypoxia of the cardiac muscle. *Mitral insufficiency* refers to an incompetent mitral valve. *Myocardial infarction* refers to death of the cardiac cells, but in angina there is no death of cells. *Coronary thrombosis* refers to an aggregation of cell elements, clotting factors, and platelets, which can lead to an occlusion of a blood vessel.

16. C) Fast heart rate

Tachycardia refers to a heart rate that is faster than normal, above 100 beats/min. Irregular heartbeat is referred to as *arrhythmia*. *Hypertension* is elevated blood pressure. *Dyspnea* is shortness of breath.

17. C) In the fifth intercostal space at the left midclavicular line

The heart's apex is between the fifth and sixth ribs at the midclavicular line, closest to the chest wall; thus, it is easiest to auscultate in this position. The median point of the sternum, sixth and seventh rib area, and third and fourth rib area cannot be accessed for auscultation because they are further above the apex.

18. The nurse identifies which of the following as a test for varicose veins that the nurse can perform?

    A. Arteriography
    B. Babinski reflex
    C. Romberg's sign
    D. Trendelenburg test

19. The nurse would prioritize care for a patient with which of the following conditions?

    A. Fractured femur
    B. Head injury
    C. Ventricular fibrillation
    D. Penetrating wound to the abdomen

20. A patient with a body mass index of 35 kg/m² is admitted for bariatric surgery. Which of the following nursing diagnoses should the nurse attend to first?

    A. Imbalanced nutrition: more than body requirements related to excessive intake in relationship to metabolic needs
    B. Impaired skin integrity related to alterations in nutritional state, immobility, excess moisture, and multiple skin folds
    C. Ineffective breathing pattern related to decreased lung expansion from obesity
    D. Chronic low self-esteem related to body size, inability to lose weight, and perceived unattractiveness

21. Which of the following symptoms are characteristic of chronic venous ulcers?

    A. The patient will feel pain and cramping in the left leg when walking.
    B. The patient will feel relief upon elevating the left leg.
    C. The patient will have a wound that is black in appearance and dry.
    D. The patient will have limited sensation to the affected area.

22. A patient with a myocardial infarction is admitted to the coronary unit. The nurse identifies that the patient is at risk for impaired tissue perfusion due to decrease in cardiac output. Which of the following assessment findings would lead the nurse to contact the healthcare provider (HCP) immediately?

    A. Blood pressure of 95/49 mmHg
    B. Heart rate of 59 beats/min
    C. A new-onset systolic murmur
    D. SpO_2 of 92% on 2 L/min oxygen via nasal prongs

23. A patient with a history of chronic renal failure is diagnosed with pericarditis after a viral infection. Which of the following nursing recommendations would help to support the patient's recovery?

    A. Take aspirin every 4 hours as needed for pain management.
    B. Engage in activity and attempt to build exercise tolerance.
    C. Use colchicine therapy to decrease inflammation.
    D. Go to the ED if any chest pain is detected.

(See answers next page.)

18. D) Trendelenburg test
The Trendelenburg test evaluates the backflow of blood through the valves. The Babinski reflex is used to determine injury to the pyramidal tracts in adults. Romberg's test is used for position and balance. Arteriography is not a test done by nurses.

19. C) Ventricular fibrillation
Ventricular fibrillation causes irreversible brain damage and death within minutes because the heart is not pumping blood. Cardiopulmonary resuscitation should be initiated immediately. The other conditions do not require such urgent treatment and assessment.

20. C) Ineffective breathing pattern related to decreased lung expansion from obesity
If the patient is at risk for ineffective breathing patterns, their respiratory status should be the primary nursing concern. Impaired skin integrity is the second most important concern because skin breakdown may lead to infection. The nurse also needs to attend to the patient's psychosocial needs and provide support. Imbalanced nutrition related to excessive intake will be managed during the patient's surgical preparation.

21. B) The patient will feel relief upon elevating the left leg.
Chronic venous ulcers result from incompetent valves of veins, typically in lower extremities, causing pressure of blood in veins to increase. This leads to blood pooling, vein wall stretching, and leaking of proteins into subcutaneous tissue. Due to the swelling, patients will feel relief when they elevate the extremity or wear compression stockings. Pain and cramping with walking is called *intermittent claudication*. This is seen in arterial ulcers. Arterial ulcers also have necrotic tissue and are black and dry. Diabetic ulcers are formed from neuropathies, which result in limited sensation to the affected areas. This can result in increased wounds and injuries.

22. C) A new-onset systolic murmur
Patients who have had a myocardial infarction are at an increased risk for rupturing the papillary muscles that secure the heart valves. A new-onset murmur is a warning sign that this may be happening. The HCP must be notified immediately, because the only treatment is valve surgery. The patient has a stable mean arterial pressure in the blood pressure provided. A low heart rate of 59 beats/min is acceptable in a patient after myocardial infarction and is likely a result of beta-blocker therapy. The patient has a stable SpO_2 on oxygen.

23. A) Take aspirin every 4 hours as needed for pain management.
Pain management is essential for recovery from pericarditis. Pain can be managed with aspirin or nonsteroidal anti-inflammatory drug (NSAID) therapy. Aspirin can be taken by patients with chronic renal failure. In some instances, other pain medications may be ordered by the healthcare provider. It is recommended that patients rest and do not engage in strenuous exercise while they are recovering. Colchicine may be given for inflammation, but should not be administered to patients with renal failure. The patient will have persistent chest pain with pericarditis; ED evaluation is not necessary.

24. A patient is admitted to a medical unit for a cerebral vascular accident (CVA). When assessing the patient, which of the following findings may be a potential risk factor for CVA?

    A. 115/74 mmHg blood pressure
    B. Noted ptosis to the right eyelid
    C. Auscultation of fine crackles in posterior lung fields
    D. Palpation of an irregular radial pulse

25. The nurse is working with a patient who had a right-brain cerebral vascular accident (CVA). Which of the following nursing diagnoses best identifies patient risk with this type of injury?

    A. Increased risk for depression related to awareness of physical deficits
    B. Impaired speech and language due to CVA
    C. At risk for impaired safety related to impulsivity
    D. Impaired comprehension related to language deficits

26. An admitted patient demonstrates signs of a cerebral vascular accident (CVA) while eating breakfast. The patient is rushed for a CT scan. The purpose of the CT scan in the early stages of a stroke is:

    A. To assess whether the brain is clear from bleeding in order to administer thrombolytic therapy for ischemic stroke.
    B. To diagnose the presence of a stroke and determine the full extent of injury to the brain.
    C. To identify potential aneurysms that may lead to hemorrhagic stroke.
    D. To reveal signs of extracranial atherosclerotic disease that may cause ischemic stroke.

27. A patient's family member is concerned that the patient is having a stroke. Which of the following nursing questions would help to complete a focused stroke assessment?

    A. Ask whether the patient is having any chest pain, confusion, or dizziness.
    B. Ask whether the patient has any sudden weakness or any sudden loss of vision or speech.
    C. Ask whether the patient has signs of fainting, low blood pressure, or a rapid heart rate.
    D. Ask whether the patient has abdominal pain, feels nauseated, or is vomiting.

28. The nurse is completing teaching regarding stroke prevention to a local community group. Which of the following health-promotion activities would help combat the major modifiable risk factors for stroke?

    A. Invite a stroke survivor to come to the group to tell their story.
    B. Organize a session focused on a ketogenic diet and its health benefits.
    C. Invite a cardiologist to speak to the group about atrial fibrillation.
    D. Conduct a session focused on smoking-cessation therapies and techniques.

(See answers next page.)

24. D) Palpation of an irregular radial pulse

Atrial fibrillation is a risk factor for CVA. One indicator that a patient may have atrial fibril-lation is an irregular pulse. The nurse would recommend an EKG to confirm the diagnosis. Hypertension is a risk factor for stroke, but this patient does not have hypertension. Ptosis to the right eyelid is most likely caused by the stroke. Auscultation of fine crackles to poste-rior lung lobes may be attributed to the patient being on bed rest.

25. C) At risk for impaired safety related to impulsivity

A patient with right-sided brain damage from a CVA will present with impulsivity and safety problems due to impaired judgment, short attention span, impaired time concepts, and a tendency to deny or minimize problems. Patients with left-sided brain injury from a CVA are at a greater risk for depression, anxiety, impaired speech or aphasia, and language deficits, and are typically cautious.

26. A) To assess whether the brain is clear from bleeding in order to administer thrombolytic therapy for ischemic stroke.

A CT scan is used to detect intracranial bleeding. In the first 4 hours after the onset of stroke symptoms, it is not possible to tell the difference between normal and ischemic areas in the brain. If the CT scan is clear for bleeding, the protocol for treating an ischemic stroke will be initiated and thrombolytic therapy will be administered. The CT will not be able to spe-cifically diagnose the extent of a stroke in early stages. An MRI is used to examine the full extent of ischemic brain injury. A noncontrast CT scan will identify bleeding in the brain. A contrast CT scan is needed to observe for aneurysms and vascular structures. Extracranial atherosclerotic disease is studied with a carotid duplex ultrasound, not a CT scan.

27. B) Ask whether the patient has any sudden weakness or any sudden loss of vision or speech.

The nurse must complete a focused assessment based on the warning signs for a stroke. This includes sudden weakness; paralysis or numbness on one or both sides of the body; sudden loss of vision in one or both eyes; sudden loss of speech; confusion; difficulty speak-ing or understanding speech; unexplained sudden dizziness; loss of balance; or a sudden or severe headache. The nurse must ascertain these risk factors to help initiate a stroke protocol and ensure that the patient receives emergency care. Chest pain, confusion, and dizziness may be related to a myocardial infarction or pulmonary embolus. Signs of fainting, low blood pressure, and a rapid heart rate could indicate a cardiac arrhythmia. Abdominal pain, nausea, or vomiting may be a sign of an intestinal obstruction, peritonitis, or appendicitis.

28. D) Conduct a session focused on smoking-cessation therapies and techniques.

A modifiable risk factor is something a patient can change. In this instance, it is smok-ing. The nurse can encourage health promotion by conducting a smoking-cessation session. Inviting a stroke survivor may help teach recognition of stroke symptoms. A ketogenic diet may affect other risk factors for stroke, such as atherosclerosis. Atrial fibrillation is a risk factor for stroke, but it would be more appropriate for the nurse to conduct the teaching session. Patient teaching is within the nurse's scope of practice.

29. The nurse is assisting a new nurse with a dressing change for a patient with an arterial ulcer. Which action by the new nurse would warrant the assisting nurse's taking immediate action?

    A. The new nurse applies a wet dressing to the wound bed and covers it with a dry dressing.
    B. The new nurse covers the wound with a dry dressing and secures it with tape.
    C. The new nurse encourages the patient to hang the leg off the bed when having pain during the dressing change.
    D. The new nurse cleanses the wound with chlorohexidine and allows it to dry.

30. A patient with an aortic dissection is prescribed a continuous infusion of nitroprusside. Which nursing intervention is of the highest priority when administering this medication?

    A. Teach the patient to report any severe abdominal pain or cramping.
    B. Complete a full patient assessment every 8 hours.
    C. Track the patient's thiocyanate levels in the chart weekly.
    D. Ensure that the patient has an arterial line or a noninvasive blood pressure cuff set for every 15 minutes.

31. A patient with coronary artery disease, type 2 diabetes mellitus, and hypertension is prescribed 50 mg of daily oral metoprolol and 5 mg of daily ramipril, both due at the same time. What information is critical to provide to the patient taking this drug therapy?

    A. It is important that metoprolol not be taken at the same time as ramipril.
    B. Metoprolol should not be taken if the patient's heart rate is under 65 beats/min.
    C. Metoprolol may mask signs of hypoglycemia. It is important to monitor blood glucose levels through the day.
    D. Metoprolol can precipitate bronchoconstriction in patients with asthma.

32. Which of the following pathogens is responsible for rheumatic fever?

    A. *Clostridium difficile*
    B. *Streptococcus*
    C. *Salmonella*
    D. *Staphylococcus*

33. The nurse is evaluating a patient's fluid balance after an ischemic stroke. Which of the following outcomes would alert the nurse to notify the healthcare provider?

    A. The patient's sodium level is 137 mEq/L.
    B. The patient's catheter bag is filled with clear urine.
    C. The patient has a bag of intravenous (IV) D5W infusing at 50 mL/hr.
    D. The patient has a blood glucose level of 120 mg/dL.

(See answers next page.)

29. A) The new nurse applies a wet dressing to the wound bed and covers it with a dry dressing.
Arterial ulcers must be kept dry. They are not to be cleansed with normal saline or soaked with wet gauze. This may cause further infection and liquid necrosis. Arterial wounds should be covered with a dry dressing to protect the area and can be secured with tape. Elevating the limb during a dressing change can cause pain. If the patient is experiencing pain, it is appropriate to dangle the leg. Chlorohexidine and povidone iodine are recommended cleansing agents for this type of wound.

30. D) Ensure that the patient has an arterial line or a noninvasive blood pressure cuff set for every 15 minutes.
Nitroprusside is a potent vasodilator given intravenously to patients with malignant hypertension or dissecting aortic aneurysms. It will decrease blood pressure in an effort to stabilize the aortic dissection. The first priority is to ensure that an accurate and frequent blood pressure is taken. An arterial line is preferred. If an arterial line is not an option, the nurse must ensure frequent and continuous monitoring of blood pressure noninvasively while nitroprusside is being administered, assessed every 15 minutes rather than waiting for a full assessment every 8 hours since sensitive changes can be quickly identified. Aortic dissection typically presents as crushing chest pain or back pain, not as lower abdominal pain or cramping. Nitroprusside breaks down into cyanide in the body; therefore, thiocyanate levels are tracked daily (not weekly).

31. C) Metoprolol may mask signs of hypoglycemia. It is important to monitor blood glucose levels through the day.
Metoprolol is a beta-blocker that inhibits the sympathetic nervous system response as well as potentially masking signs of hypoglycemia. Patients with diabetes taking this therapy should engage in a routine of blood glucose testing to ensure their safety. Beta-blockers and angiotensin-converting enzyme (ACE) inhibitors can be taken at the same time because they exert different effects on the heart and complement each other by increasing myocardial contractility while decreasing systemic vascular resistance. Typically, a patient will hold off on taking metoprolol if the heart rate is under 60 beats/min. Propranolol is a common nonselective beta-blocker and can cause bronchospasm in patients with asthma because it inhibits beta 1 and 2.

32. B) *Streptococcus*
Acute rheumatic fever is a complication that occurs as a delayed sequela (usually after 2–3 weeks) of group A streptococcal pharyngitis. *Clostridium difficile* is associated with infections of the intestines, salmonella is a foodborne bacteria leading to gastrointestinal dysfunction, and *Staphylococcus* is typically linked to skin infections.

33. C) The patient has a bag of intravenous (IV) D5W infusing at 50 mL/hr.
The nurse would need to notify the healthcare provider if a hypertonic IV solution was administered to the patient because this solution may potentially pull water into the brain tissue and cause cerebral edema. The patient should also be monitored for low sodium levels because they are a sign of fluid overload; however, the sodium level is normal in this case. Patients may have large amounts of clear urine after a stroke. Hyperglycemia can also cause further brain damage, but the glucose level is normal.

34. A patient is ordered telemetry monitoring after surgery. The telemetry nurse calls up to the unit to report that the patient's rhythm is a sinus bradycardia at 37 beats/min. What nursing priority should be evaluated at this time?

    A. Prepare to administer atropine to the patient.
    B. Ask the patient whether they feel short of breath or dizzy.
    C. Reassess the patient's heart rate by palpating the radial pulse.
    D. Reassess the patient's blood pressure.

35. The nurse is evaluating a teaching session for a patient with an implantable cardioverter-defibrillator (ICD). Which of the following patient statements demonstrates knowledge of maintaining personal safety with this device?

    A. "I should have my ICD checked every year with an interrogator-programmer device."
    B. "It is important that I lie down when the ICD fires."
    C. "The ICD device means my family members do not have to do cardiopulmonary resuscitation (CPR)."
    D. "I will be able to drive now that the ICD is in place."

36. A case manager is evaluating a patient with congestive heart failure who is in the hospital. Which of the following outcomes would demonstrate an improvement in the patient's condition?

    A. The patient has fine crackles to the posterior left lower lung lobe.
    B. The patient is adhering to a fluid restriction of 1.5 L/d.
    C. The patient has a beta natriuretic peptide (BNP) level within the normal therapeutic range.
    D. The patient has a blood pressure of 104/63 mmHg.

37. A patient is discharged home after having infective endocarditis. Which of the following outcomes would demonstrate an improvement in the patient's condition?

    A. The patient experiences intermittent chest pain that resolves with rest.
    B. The patient remains afebrile with no signs of malaise or chills.
    C. The patient no longer has a pericardial rub upon auscultation of the heart.
    D. The patient notes decreased anxiety.

38. A patient is experiencing periodic episodes of paroxysmal supraventricular tachycardia (PSVT) associated with stress. How can the nurse empower the patient while developing self-care strategies for managing PSVT?

    A. Teach the patient three different types of vasovagal maneuvers to try when they have an episode of PSVT at home.
    B. Help the patient access online stress reduction techniques.
    C. Ensure that the patient understands that PSVT is a medical emergency requiring an immediate trip to the ED.
    D. Encourage the patient to rest during an episode of PSVT until the arrhythmia resolves.

(See answers next page.)

34. D) Reassess the patient's blood pressure.

The nurse will need to reassess if the patient is symptomatic with the bradycardia. A nursing priority is to take the patient's blood pressure to gain objective data. During that time, the nurse will also observe for shortness of breath, confusion, dizziness, syncope, loss of consciousness, or swelling in the extremities. The nurse does not need to reassess the radial pulse because the telemetry monitoring is a better indicator. It would not be appropriate to administer atropine until the patient is assessed, and a healthcare provider's order would be needed for this action.

35. B) "It is important that I lie down when the ICD fires."

An ICD is for patients who have survived sudden cardiac death, have spontaneous sustained ventricular tachycardia, have syncope with ventricular tachycardia during electrophysiological studies, or are at high risk for future ventricular dysrhythmias. To promote safety, the patient should lie down when the device fires. The device is checked every 2 to 3 months with an interrogator-programmer device. Family members are recommended to learn CPR. The patient with an ICD can drive only if medically cleared to do so by the healthcare provider.

36. C) The patient has a beta natriuretic peptide (BNP) level within the normal therapeutic range.

The case manager is looking for a clinical indicator for the improvement of heart failure. This would be best represented in a normal BNP level. Fine crackles to the posterior lung fields demonstrate that the acute episode may not be resolved. Even though the patient is adhering to fluid restriction, it is not an indicator of improvement; it does demonstrate adherence to health practices. The patient's blood pressure is within an acceptable range.

37. B) The patient remains afebrile with no signs of malaise or chills.

Infective endocarditis (or bacterial endocarditis) is an infection of the heart valves or the endocardial surface of the heart. Because this condition is treated with antibiotic therapy, absence of an infection and no fever would be indicators of improvement. Pericarditis is associated with intermittent chest pain and a pericardial rub. Anxiety may be a factor in any cardiac disease condition. Fever is the main measure for endocarditis and should be resolved.

38. A) Teach the patient three different types of vasovagal maneuvers to try when he has an episode of PSVT at home.

PSVT originates in an ectopic focus anywhere above the bifurcation of the bundle of His. *Paroxysmal* means it starts and stops abruptly and is treated through vasovagal maneuvers and drug therapy. Having the patient access online resources for stress may help prevent PSVT, but it does not provide self-care strategies for managing it. The patient does not have to go to the ED unless there is evidence of dizziness/fainting, the patient is unable to vasovagally maneuver out of the rhythm, or the patient is unconscious.

39. Two nurses attempted to mobilize a patient with a left-brain stroke using a sit-to-stand lift. During the transfer, the patient fell and an incident report was filed. What may be a further question by the quality officer after reviewing the submitted incident report?

   A. "Did you assess the patient's ability to understand directions?"
   B. "Did you assess the patient for any left-sided neglect?"
   C. "Were you aware if the patient had any spatial-perceptual deficits?"
   D. "Did the patient become impulsive and rush the process?"

40. A patient in cardiac arrest is currently being treated by the code team. The primary nurse was on break when the code was started. It is noted that the patient has an advance directive which states that no advanced measures or cardiopulmonary resuscitation (CPR) should be given. What is the nurse's professional role in this situation?

   A. The nurse must dismiss the code team and bring a copy of the patient's advance directive.
   B. Once CPR is started, the code team cannot stop until it has been determined to be medically futile.
   C. The nurse should contact the hospital's legal department on how to proceed with this situation.
   D. The nurse will need to contact the patient's family for guidance.

41. The nurse is assigned to a patient with infective endocarditis. The nurse refuses to care for the patient because of a history of drug abuse. What can the nurse be charged with if the nurse does not accept this assignment?

   A. Assault
   B. Malpractice
   C. Negligence
   D. Abandonment

42. A patient is admitted to a medical unit for a non–ST-elevation myocardial infarction (NSTEMI). Which of the following nursing interventions will help maintain patient safety by decreasing myocardial oxygen demand?

   A. Put on the bed alarm in case the patient falls out of bed.
   B. Ensure that the patient is on bed rest for the first 24 hours.
   C. Use a sit-to-stand lift when mobilizing the patient to the toilet.
   D. Increase the patient's oxygen to maintain SpO_2 of 100%.

(See answers next page.)

39. A) "Did you assess the patient's ability to understand directions?"

Patients with left-brain injuries have right-sided involvement (e.g., right hemiplegia). They may also have expressive, receptive, or global aphasia impairing their ability to understand directions, which may have led to the fall. Patients with right-brain injuries have left-sided involvement (e.g., left hemiplegia or spatial-perceptual deficits) and often demonstrate impulsivity.

40. A) The nurse must dismiss the code team and bring a copy of the patient's advance directive.

The nurse is responsible for ensuring that the code team is aware of the advance directive. It is a legal document that guides care. Decisions for care once a code has been started will be determined by this document. If it is deemed that the patient did not wish to have CPR, it will be stopped. This situation is too urgent to wait for the hospital's legal team to respond. The nurse should work from the advance directive and not the family's input.

41. D) Abandonment

The nurse cannot refuse a patient assignment unless the nurse's safety is at risk (e.g., the nurse has a medical condition that may worsen if exposed to a particular patient population). The nurse could be charged with patient abandonment (leaving the patient) if the nurse refused care. Negligence is an act or omission that deviates from the regular standard of care. Malpractice is a form of negligence that results in harm to the patient. *Assault* refers to physically, mentally, or emotionally harming a patient.

42. B) Ensure that the patient is on bed rest for the first 24 hours.

The nurse will decrease the patient's activity and encourage rest for the first 24 hours by placing the patient on bed rest. The patient does not require a bed alarm or sit-to-stand lift because the question stem does not indicate that this patient is at risk for falling or that the patient has mobility issues. The patient may have the oxygen increased when mobilizing, but it is not necessary to maintain an SpO_2 of 100%, which may cause oxygen toxicity if used for prolonged periods.

Hematological System

1. A patient diagnosed with macrocytic anemia requires therapy. Which of the following nursing statements describes to the patient how this therapy is administered?

   A. "Your healthcare provider will need to evaluate whether you are having any internal bleeding."

   B. "You will be required to have an intramuscular injection of vitamin B12 once a week through the outpatient clinic."

   C. "You will be required to take erythropoietin injections once a week."

   D. "It is important that you increase the amount of iron in your diet and take iron supplements daily."

2. The nurse assesses a patient in septic shock and finds extensive petechiae, lower left leg pain, and hematuria. Which laboratory findings would alert the nurse that the patient may have disseminated intravascular coagulopathy (DIC)?

   A. Prolonged partial thromboplastin time (PTT), prolonged prothrombin time (PT), and elevated D-dimer

   B. Decreased hemoglobin, increased platelets, and increased neutrophils

   C. Decreased international normalized ratio (INR), prolonged PTT, and increased C-reactive protein

   D. Increased white blood cell count, increased hematocrit, and increased mean corpuscular volume

3. The nurse is providing dietary teaching for a patient with hemochromatosis. Which of the following patient statements would indicate that more teaching is required?

   A. "I typically eat yogurt and berries for breakfast with coffee or tea."

   B. "I often snack on nuts in between meals."

   C. "My favorite meal is sushi with a citrus salad and broccoli."

   D. "On weekends I enjoy bacon, eggs, and toast."

4. A patient with hemophilia is admitted to the ED with a laceration to the left lower arm. What should be the nurse's first step in treating this patient?

   A. Draw bloodwork to check the partial thromboplastin time (PTT), platelet count, and factor assays.

   B. Encourage the patient to hold the extremity above the level of the heart.

   C. Provide firm pressure to the injury site until the bleeding subsides.

   D. Notify the healthcare provider and prepare for factor replacement therapy.

1. B) "You will be required to have an intramuscular injection of vitamin B12 once a week through the outpatient clinic."

Megaloblastic anemias result from vitamin B12 and folate deficiencies. In vitamin B12 deficiencies, patients are missing an intrinsic factor in the small intestines, which transforms vitamin B12 into the vascular component. Therefore, they are unable to absorb B12 through the gastrointestinal tract, and it must be given via the parenteral route. Evaluation for active bleeding is associated with conditions that incur blood loss. Red blood cells would be normochromic in these conditions. Erythropoietin injections are for anemia related to chronic renal failure. Iron-deficiency anemias require iron replacement; cells are microcytic in this type of anemia.

2. A) Prolonged partial thromboplastin time (PPT), prolonged prothrombin time (PT), and elevated D-dimer

Screening tests for DIC include PT (prolonged), PTT (prolonged), activated partial thromboplastic time (aPTT; prolonged), thrombin time (prolonged), fibrinogen (reduced), platelet (reduced), D-dimer (elevated), protein C (reduced), protein S (reduced), and antithrombin III time (reduced).

3. C) "My favorite meal is sushi with a citrus salad and broccoli."

Patients living with hemochromatosis do not excrete iron from the body. This may be due to a C282Y gene mutation or linked to another hematologic disorder. This iron overload can cause severe complications such as liver failure. Patients must avoid vitamin C, iron supplements, uncooked seafood, and iron-rich foods in their diet. Calcium-rich foods, coffee, tea, nuts, and egg yolks are known to block iron absorption and are recommended.

4. D) Notify the healthcare provider and prepare for factor replacement therapy.

Factor replacement therapy must be initiated immediately and will continue for up to 72 hours for a minor injury. The patient has known hemophilia, so it would consume precious time to draw laboratory blood work as a first priority. The patient may hold the extremity above heart level and apply pressure, but because of the limited clotting factors, the bleeding will continue. Factor replacement is the only intervention that will stabilize such a patient.

5. A patient is experiencing drenching night sweats and unexplained weight loss. Based on the nurse's knowledge of B symptoms in Hodgkin's lymphoma, what is a priority patient assessment?

   A. Assess the patient's temperature and notify the healthcare provider if the patient is febrile.
   B. Assess the patient for signs of superficial or systemic bleeding.
   C. Palpate the patient's lymph nodes and assess for enlargement or pain.
   D. Auscultate the patient's lung fields for stridor, abnormal breath sounds, and decreased air entry.

6. A patient is admitted to an acute care setting for treatment for myelodysplastic syndrome (MDS). Which of the following medication orders would alert the nurse to call the healthcare provider to clarify the order?

   A. Prednisone 10 mg orally twice a day
   B. Aspirin 80 mg orally daily
   C. Allopurinol 100 mg orally three times a day
   D. Furosemide 40 mg intravenously daily

7. The nurse finds a patient with multiple myeloma unconscious and seizing. Which laboratory value associated with this condition is essential to confirm during this clinical emergency?

   A. Magnesium 2.0 mEq/L
   B. Sodium 146 mEq/L
   C. Potassium 5.0 mEq/L
   D. Calcium 15 mg/dL

8. A patient undergoing chemotherapy is diagnosed with neutropenia. What is the patient at risk for with this condition?

   A. Infection
   B. Bleeding
   C. Immobility
   D. Pain

9. A patient with acute myeloid leukemia (AML) asks the nurse why they feel tired all the time. What is the best nursing response?

   A. "It may be helpful to increase the amount of folate in your diet to increase your energy levels."
   B. "It is important that you take frequent rest periods during the day to preserve your energy levels."
   C. "Anemia is a common complication of AML. Let's check your hemoglobin levels in the chart."
   D. "It is very stressful living with leukemia. Would you like to talk more about how you are feeling?"

(See answers next page.)

5. A) Assess the patient's temperature and notify the healthcare provider if the patient is febrile.

B symptoms are linked to an unfavorable prognosis in Hodgkin's lymphoma. B symptoms include drenching night sweats, unexplained weight loss of more than 10% of total body weight in a 6-month period, and unexplained fever of 100°F or higher. Lymph node enlargement is not painful in this condition. Bleeding occurs from pancytopenia in advanced stages. Respiratory distress suggests progressive mediastinal involvement of the disease.

6. B) Aspirin 80 mg orally daily

Patients with MDS are at an increased risk of bleeding. Antiplatelet drugs, such as aspirin, should be avoided. Prednisone is administered to help provide immunosuppression in MDS. Allopurinol helps to decrease uric acid levels. Furosemide promotes renal excretion of calcium. Uremia and hypercalcemia are complications related to MDS.

7. D) Calcium 15 mg/dL

Hypercalcemia is associated with multiple myeloma. This is due to bone destruction associated with increased cytokines present in the condition. Hypercalcemia can lead to confusion, seizures, and coma. The magnesium level is normal. The sodium level is slightly elevated but not at a clinical level at which neurologic symptoms would occur. The potassium level is normal.

8. A) Infection

Neutropenia is a decreased count in neutrophils. This puts the patient at an increased risk for infection. The most common cause of neutropenia is use of chemotherapeutic and immunosuppressant drugs. Bleeding risk occurs with a low platelet count. This may result from chemotherapy or the form of cancer. Immobility may be due to weakness or pain from the cancer. Cancer pain results from pressure on body organs or nerves.

9. C) "Anemia is a common complication of AML. Let's check your hemoglobin levels in the chart."

The patient is asking about potential causes of their fatigue. In AML, pancytopenia occurs due to the increased production of myeloid blast cells. This results in decreased red blood cells, lymphocytes, and platelets. The patient may be experiencing anemia (decreased red blood cells). The nurse should provide this education and check the patient's laboratory levels.

10. A client with suspected leukemia is scheduled for a bone marrow biopsy. Which nursing statement about the procedure provides the most accurate teaching?

A. "You will be provided with general anesthesia during the procedure."

B. "You may experience pain at the site of the biopsy and will need to be monitored for any bleeding after the procedure."

C. "You will be unable to shower for 5 days after the procedure."

D. "It is important that you immobilize the site of the biopsy for a week after the procedure."

11. A 72-year-old patient is diagnosed with chronic lymphoid leukemia (CLL) after routine blood testing. The patient did not have any previous symptoms. Which of the following nursing statements best describes indications for chemotherapy in CLL?

A. "The healthcare provider will initiate chemotherapy if you start experiencing adverse symptoms related to this disease condition."

B. "It is important for you to start chemotherapy as soon as possible. Your healthcare provider will be in contact with you."

C. "This condition can be treated with a medication called *imatinib*."

D. "You will need to monitor for signs of infection prior to starting chemotherapy because this condition will decrease your white blood cell count."

12. A patient with chronic myeloid leukemia (CML) has splenomegaly, a common complication associated with the condition. Which of the following nursing diagnoses aligns with splenomegaly?

A. Upper right-sided abdominal discomfort related to pain

B. Increased fatigue related to decreased exercise capacity

C. Increased bone and joint discomfort related to body position

D. Decreased nutritional intake related to early satiety

13. A patient with a low hemoglobin level presents with fatigue, palpitations, and a smooth tongue. Which type of anemia is the patient likely experiencing?

A. Anemia associated with chronic renal failure

B. Iron-deficiency anemia (microcytic anemia)

C. Vitamin B12 and folate deficiency anemia (macrocytic anemia)

D. Anemia related to acute blood loss

14. A patient with acute myeloid leukemia (AML) has a nursing diagnosis of "at risk for infection due to pancytopenia from chemotherapy." Which of the following nursing interventions will help to prevent infection?

A. Ensure that the patient receives irradiated blood products.

B. Recommend medications via the oral route when possible.

C. Increase the patient's daily caloric intake to meet metabolic demands related to the disease condition.

D. Put the patient in reverse isolation using airborne precautions.

(See answers next page.)

10. B) "You may experience pain at the site of the biopsy and will need to be monitored for any bleeding after the procedure."

A bone marrow biopsy removes a portion of the bone marrow via a slender needle. The patient may experience pain at the site and will be monitored for bleeding from the site before the patient is discharged from the hospital. The procedure does not include general anesthesia. It is recommended that patients not get the biopsy site wet, but they are still permitted to shower. The site of the biopsy need not be immobilized; rather, the site should be rested for a day after the procedure. Vigorous exercise or heavy lifting should be avoided.

11. A) "The healthcare provider will initiate chemotherapy if you start experiencing adverse symptoms related to this disease condition."

About 25% to 50% of patients diagnosed with CLL have no symptoms. Because this condition commonly appears in late adulthood, treatment with chemotherapy is not initiated until symptoms appear. Imatinib is a medication used in chronic myeloid leukemia (CML), not CLL. CLL is a condition in which there is an increased production of lymphocytes.

12. D) Decreased nutritional intake related to early satiety

Splenomegaly is associated with decreased appetite and early satiety. This may result in decreased nutritional intake in patients with CML. Abdominal discomfort and pain would present on the left side of the abdomen. Increased fatigue and decreased exercise capacity may result from anemia associated with CML. Increased bone and joint pain may result from blast crisis but are not symptoms of splenomegaly.

13. B) Iron-deficiency anemia (microcytic anemia)

The patient may be experiencing iron-deficiency anemia. Signs related to this condition include pica (abnormal food cravings), smooth tongue, fatigue, low serum ferritin levels, low hemoglobin levels, and pale skin/mucous membranes. Anemia from chronic renal failure presents with classic anemia symptoms (e.g., fatigue, weakness, dizziness) but will also show signs of albumin in the urine. Vitamin B12 and folate deficiency anemias may present with confusion, fatigue, and tingling in the hands or feet. Anemia related to acute blood loss results in hypotension, tachycardia, and signs of myocardia ischemia (e.g., chest pain).

14. B) Recommend medications via the oral route when possible.

Infection in AML results from low neutrophils and lymphocytes. Pancytopenia is a decrease in red blood cells, platelets, and lymphocytes. The nurse should decrease the amount of invasive procedures related to medication administration, such as injections. The oral route is the least invasive method of administration. Irradiated blood products are recommended to prevent graft-versus-host disease. Increasing a patient's metabolic demands and nutritional intake may promote healing, but it will not directly prevent infection. Patients receiving chemotherapy who have neutropenia do not show better outcomes from reverse isolation. Airborne precautions are not implemented in this instance.

15. A patient is admitted to the medical unit with anemia of unknown origin. The nurse completes an initial assessment, formulates a nursing diagnosis, and creates a care plan. Which of the following symptoms would require immediate reassessment by the nurse?

    A. The patient has 90/60 mmHg blood pressure.
    B. The patient has a blood oxygen saturation level (SpO_2) level of 89% on room air.
    C. The patient is demonstrating confusion and chest pain.
    D. The patient has gingival bleeding and thinning hair.

16. The nurse is evaluating self-care practices for a patient with hemochromatosis. Which of the following patient statements would alert the nurse to reinforce the previous teaching?

    A. "I will need to go for a therapeutic phlebotomy each week for 2 to 3 years or until my iron stores are depleted."
    B. "I will need to report any right-upper-quadrant abdominal pain or signs of jaundice to my healthcare professional."
    C. "It is important that I avoid foods high in vitamin C."
    D. "I will limit my iron intake through my diet, but I will still be able to drink alcohol in moderation."

(See answers next page.)

15. C) The patient is demonstrating confusion and chest pain.

The patient may be demonstrating signs of a myocardial infarction as a result of the anemia and hypoxia. This should prompt the nurse to call the healthcare provider and redirect the plan of care. The blood pressure has a low systolic pressure but a mean arterial pressure (MAP) of 70 mmHg. This is a stable blood pressure. The patient is expected to have a decreased blood oxygen saturation level (SpO_2); the nurse can apply oxygen therapy. Gingival bleeding and thinning hair are signs of chronic anemia.

16. D) "I will limit my iron intake through my diet, but I will still be able to drink alcohol in moderation."

In order to prevent further liver damage in hemochromatosis, it is recommended to limit alcohol intake. The patient will need to go for a therapeutic phlebotomy to remove 500 mL of blood each week for 2 to 3 years or until the iron load is decreased. The patient should report any signs of liver dysfunction, which may include right-upper-quadrant abdominal pain, jaundice, or dark amber urine. The patient should avoid foods high in vitamin C because they aid in iron absorption in the body.

Endocrine System

1. The nurse is preparing to apply an external pacemaker to a patient with an endocrinology disorder. For which patient is the nurse most likely implementing this procedure?

   A. A patient with thyroid storm
   B. A patient with pheochromocytoma
   C. A patient with myxedema coma
   D. A patient with Cushing's syndrome

2. The nurse was notified that a patient with tremors, tachycardia, and intolerance to heat has a low thyroid-stimulating hormone (TSH) level. The nurse understands that the patient has a diagnosis of:

   A. Hyperthyroidism.
   B. Hypothyroidism.
   C. Hypoparathyroidism.
   D. Hyperparathyroidism.

3. The nurse is teaching a patient about hypothyroidism. Which of the following statements should the nurse include in the teaching plan?

   A. Increase calorie intake.
   B. Increase home temperature.
   C. Take levothyroxine at night.
   D. Limit fiber intake.

4. The nurse is caring for a patient with type 1 diabetes. The patient takes isophane (neutral protamine Hagedorn [NPH]) insulin at night and reports an elevation of blood glucose in the morning. To identify the Somogyi effect, the nurse anticipates that which of the following actions is needed?

   A. Increase the NPH units at night.
   B. Obtain a blood glucose reading at 3:00 a.m.
   C. Decrease food intake at night.
   D. Take an extra dose of NPH insulin in the morning.

5. The nurse is teaching a patient about diabetes control. The nurse should teach the patient that proper diabetes management happens when the hemoglobin A1C is below:

   A. 10%
   B. 9%
   C. 8%
   D. 7%

(See answers next page.)

1. C) A patient with myxedema coma
An external pacemaker is applied to a patient with a slow heart rate. A patient with a myxedema coma has extreme bradycardia. Patients with pheochromocytoma, thyroid storm, and Cushing's syndrome have tachycardia and do not need an external pacemaker.

2. A) Hyperthyroidism
Patients with hyperthyroidism exhibit tachycardia, intolerance to heat, and low TSH. Hypothyroidism shows high TSH. Parathyroid disorders show problems with blood calcium levels.

3. B) Increase home temperature.
Patients with hypothyroidism suffer from intolerance to cold. By increasing home temperature, they will feel more comfortable. Levothyroxine is taken in the morning. Patients should decrease calorie intake and increase fiber intake.

4. B) Obtain a blood glucose reading at 3:00 a.m.
A patient with the Somogyi effect will have rebound hyperglycemia in the morning due to hypoglycemia at 3:00 a.m. The nurse should take a blood glucose level reading at that time. Increasing insulin units or decreasing food intake at night will cause more hypoglycemia. An extra dosage in the morning will not change the hyperglycemia.

5. D) 7%
A patient with well-managed diabetes should have a hemoglobin A1C below 7%.

6. The nurse was informed that a patient with a positive Trousseau sign has a calcium level of 4 mg/dL. The nurse recognized that the patient has:

   A. Hyperthyroidism.
   B. Hypoparathyroidism.
   C. Hyperparathyroidism.
   D. Hypothyroidism.

7. A nurse is caring for a patient with syndrome of inappropriate antidiuretic hormone secretion (SIADH). Which of the following assessments could indicate that the prescribed therapy is effective?

   A. The patient reports increased shortness of breath.
   B. The patient's urine specific gravity is increased.
   C. The patient's weight is decreased.
   D. The urine output is decreased.

8. The nurse is assessing a patient with diabetes insipidus. Which of the following assessment findings supports that diagnosis?

   A. Crackles in the lungs
   B. Increased weight
   C. Increased urinary output
   D. Distention of the jugular veins

9. The nurse is to administer prescribed nasal desmopressin to a patient with diabetes insipidus. Which assessment finding will require immediate follow-up by the nurse?

   A. The patient has sinusitis.
   B. The patient has an increased blood glucose level.
   C. The patient has an increase in urine osmolality.
   D. The patient's appetite is decreased.

10. The nurse is caring for a patient with diabetic ketoacidosis. Which of the following nursing diagnoses should the nurse include in the plan of care?

    A. Impaired tissue perfusion
    B. Fluid volume deficit
    C. Nutrition more than body requirements
    D. Activity intolerance

11. Which of the following is essential to consider before administering insulin lispro?

    A. Make sure the insulin is cold.
    B. Food must be placed by the patient's bedside.
    C. A patent intravenous (IV) is present.
    D. The nurse is to review the latest Hb A1C.

(See answers next page.)

6. B) Hypoparathyroidism.

Patients with hypoparathyroidism exhibit a positive Trousseau sign, which indicates low calcium levels in the blood.

7. C) The patient's weight is decreased.

In SIADH, the patient retains fluids due to increased antidiuretic hormone. If the patient's weight decreases, the therapy has been effective. The other choices indicate that the disorder is not improving.

8. C) Increased urinary output

Patients with diabetes insipidus have a decreased antidiuretic hormone, which causes an increase in the urinary output. The other choices support the diagnosis of syndrome of inappropriate antidiuretic hormone secretion (SIADH).

9. A) The patient has sinusitis.

A patient with sinusitis who is receiving nasal desmopressin will not absorb the medication. The nurse should report the situation to have the route changed. Having an increase in the blood glucose level, an increase in urine osmolality, or a decrease in appetite would not require further follow-up for administration of the drug.

10. B) Fluid volume deficit

Patients with diabetic ketoacidosis have severe hyperglycemia. Symptoms of hyperglycemia include polyuria, polydipsia, polyphagia, and weight loss. A nursing diagnosis of fluid volume deficit is important to include in the plan of care. Impaired tissue perfusion is a diagnosis for circulatory problems. Activity intolerance is more appropriate for respiratory conditions. Nutrition, more than body requirements, applies to low weight.

11. B) Food must be placed by the patient's bedside.

Insulin lispro is a rapid-acting insulin that usually starts working 5 minutes after administration. Food must be placed next to the patient's bedside. Insulin should be administered at room temperature. It is given subcutaneously and does not require a review of the Hb A1C.

12. A nurse is teaching a patient newly diagnosed with type 1 diabetes. The patient tells the nurse, "I will keep the insulin I am using in the fridge for longer use." Which of the following nursing diagnoses is the most appropriate to include in the plan of care?

   A. Altered mental status related to disease process
   B. Ineffective denial related to new diagnosis
   C. Hopelessness
   D. Knowledge deficit about disease management

13. The nurse is teaching a patient with type 2 diabetes about safety concerns while using canagliflozin. Which of the following safety measures should the nurse teach to the patient?

   A. Take your blood pressure once a week.
   B. Check your weight periodically.
   C. Notify your healthcare provider if you experience polyuria and polydipsia.
   D. Follow up with a liver function test occasionally.

14. The nurse is preparing an educational in-service about Addison's disease. Which information should the nurse include in the teaching plan?

   A. Patients will be prone to hyperglycemia.
   B. Patients will need to take potassium supplements.
   C. Patients will need to take corticosteroids.
   D. Patients will develop hypertension.

15. The nurse is assessing a patient with Addison's disease. Which physical assessment findings should the nurse anticipate?

   A. Bruises
   B. Central obesity
   C. Tanned skin
   D. Exophthalmos

16. The nurse is reviewing laboratory data for a patient with syndrome of inappropriate antidiuretic hormone secretion (SIADH). Which of the following results should the nurse anticipate?

   A. Decreased sodium level
   B. Decreased urine osmolality
   C. Decreased potassium level
   D. Increased serum osmolality

17. The nurse is collecting a sample to help diagnose a patient with pheochromocytoma. Which sample should the nurse collect?

   A. A sputum sample
   B. A blood sample
   C. A 24-hour urine collection
   D. A nasal swab

(See answers next page.)

12. D) Knowledge deficit about disease management

Opened insulin should be kept at room temperature for 28 days to diminish irritation to injection site. The patient is showing knowledge deficit about their disease management. Altered mental status is not applicable because the patient demonstrates a logical yet incorrect mental process. The patient is not in denial or hopeless; therefore, those diagnoses are not appropriate.

13. C) Notify your healthcare provider if you experience polyuria and polydipsia.

Canagliflozin is associated with diabetic ketoacidosis. Signs of ketoacidosis include polyuria and polydipsia. It is essential for the nurse to teach the patient to notify the healthcare provider if these symptoms occur. Canagliflozin does not affect blood pressure, liver function test results, or weight.

14. C) Patients will need to take corticosteroids.

Patients with Addison's disease will need to take corticosteroids to replace the missing adrenal production. These patients may have hypoglycemia, rather than hyperglycemia, due to the deficiency in cortisol balance. Calcium is generally not affected in Addison's disease. A deficiency of aldosterone results in large amounts of sodium being excreted, leading to low sodium levels while retaining potassium, resulting in low blood pressure.

15. C) Tanned skin

Patients with Addison's disease will have tanned skin. Bruises and central obesity are seen in patients with Cushing's syndrome. Exophthalmos is seen in hyperthyroidism.

16. A) Decreased sodium level

Patients with SIADH retain water, causing diluted sodium levels. Potassium is not affected in SIADH. Patients develop decreased serum osmolality and increased urine osmolality.

17. C) A 24-hour urine collection

Pheochromocytoma is diagnosed by the level of catecholamines in the urine. A 24-hour urine collection is needed to measure catecholamine levels. Nasal swabs, blood samples, or sputum samples are not used to diagnose the condition.

18. The nurse is reviewing laboratory data for a patient with uncontrolled advanced type 2 diabetes. Which of the following results should the nurse anticipate?

    A. Negative levels of glucose in the urine
    B. Microproteinuria in the urine
    C. Hemoglobin A1C of 6%
    D. Fasting blood glucose levels below 130 mg/dL

19. The nurse is preparing an educational in-service program about hyperparathyroidism. Which information should the nurse include in the teaching plan?

    A. Patients have low calcium levels.
    B. Patients are at risk for kidney stones.
    C. Patients have increased phosphorus levels.
    D. Patients will have a positive Trousseau sign.

20. The nurse is teaching a newly diagnosed type 1 diabetic patient about the sick-days rules. What should the nurse include in the teaching plan?

    A. Double the doses of oral antidiabetes medication.
    B. Decrease insulin units.
    C. Check urine for ketones.
    D. Decrease fluid intake.

21. The nurse understands that a patient with hypoparathyroidism will have:

    A. A low serum calcium level.
    B. Nausea and vomiting.
    C. Confusion.
    D. Kidney stones.

22. The nurse is caring for a patient with type 2 diabetes. Which prescription will the nurse administer to the patient?

    A. Levothyroxine
    B. Enoxaparin
    C. Empagliflozin
    D. Hydrocortisone

23. The nurse is caring for a patient with hypothyroidism. Which assessment finding indicates that the prescribed therapy has been effective?

    A. Slow mental process
    B. Pulse of 80 beats/min
    C. Weight gain of 4 lb in 1 week
    D. Cold skin

(See answers next page.)

18. B) Microproteinuria in the urine
A diabetic patient with uncontrolled sugar will have glucosuria, microproteinuria, hemo-globin A1C more than 9%, and elevated levels of fasting blood glucose.

19. B) Patients are at risk for kidney stones.
A patient with hyperparathyroidism will have increased serum calcium levels, which will increase the risk for kidney stone formation. Phosphorus levels will be decreased. Trousseau sign is positive in hypoparathyroidism, not hyperparathyroidism.

20. C) Check urine for ketones.
A patient with type 1 diabetes needs to check urine for ketones because the sickness increases blood glucose levels and can lead the patient to diabetic ketoacidosis. Type 1 diabetes is not treated with oral medications. Instead, fluids should be increased during sickness, and insulin units should correspondingly increase.

21. A) A low serum calcium level.
A patient with hypoparathyroidism has low serum calcium levels. Nausea and vomiting, presence of kidney stones, and confusion are often seen in hypercalcemia.

22. C) Empagliflozin
Empagliflozin is a sodium-glucose co-transporter 2 (SGLT2) inhibitor that causes elimina-tion of sugar in the urine. The other medications are not used in type 2 diabetes.

23. B) Pulse of 80 beats/min
The patient with hypothyroidism that is improving will show a normal heart rate. The other conditions represent signs and symptoms of the disease.

24. The nurse is caring for a patient with hyperthyroidism. Which prescription does the nurse anticipate administering?

    A. Levothyroxine
    B. Metoprolol
    C. Metformin
    D. Vasopressin

25. The nurse is caring for a post-thyroidectomy patient who arrived to the postanesthesia care unit (PACU) 15 minutes ago. Which of the following interventions should the nurse implement?

    A. Keep the patient in the supine position.
    B. Check the patient's vital signs every 2 hours.
    C. Keep the patient in a semi-Fowler's position.
    D. Administer a dose of methimazole.

26. The nurse is evaluating the therapeutic response for a patient receiving desmopressin for diabetes insipidus (DI). Which assessment finding indicates a therapeutic response?

    A. Increased urinary output
    B. Increased serum osmolality
    C. Increased urine specific gravity
    D. Increased thirst

27. The nurse is helping a patient with hyperthyroidism make dietary choices. Overall, the best choice would be:

    A. Calorie-rich meals.
    B. Meals with high fiber.
    C. Low-calorie diet.
    D. Meals high in fat.

28. The nurse is planning an in-service for a group of young adults about preventing type 2 diabetes. Which information related to prevention of type 2 diabetes is essential to include in the teaching?

    A. Eat a diet with no carbohydrates.
    B. Keep your body mass index (BMI) between 18 and 24.
    C. Limit your salt intake.
    D. Exercise twice a week.

29. A nurse is reviewing labs for a patient diagnosed with hypoparathyroidism. The nurse could expect alterations in which electrolytes?

    A. Sodium and potassium
    B. Chloride and magnesium
    C. Phosphorus and sodium
    D. Phosphorus and calcium

(See answers next page.)

24. B) Metoprolol
Metoprolol is used to control the sympathetic symptoms associated with increased thyroid hormones. Levothyroxine is used for hypothyroidism, metformin is used for diabetes, and vasopressin is used for diabetes insipidus.

25. C) Keep the patient in a semi-Fowler's position.
Post-thyroidectomy patients need to be kept in the semi-Fowler's position to prevent suture separation. Keeping the patient in the supine position is not indicated. Vital signs should be taken every 15 minutes in the PACU. Methimazole is used to block the excess thyroid hormone. Once the thyroid is removed, methimazole is no longer needed.

26. C) Increased urine specific gravity
A patient with DI who is taking desmopressin should respond to this medication with an increase in urine specific gravity because it is indicated as antidiuretic replacement therapy. An increase in serum osmolality, an increase in urinary output, and a increase in thirst are not therapeutic responses seen with desmopressin therapy for DI.

27. A) Calorie-rich meals.
Patients with hyperthyroidism burn calories at a high rate, resulting in weight loss, so a calorie-rich diet will help them gain weight. Meals with high fiber may result in an increase in diarrhea. A low-calorie diet would not provide adequate nutrition for this patient. A diet high in fat is not recommended.

28. B) Keep your body mass index (BMI) between 18 and 24.
To prevent type 2 diabetes, maintain a BMI between 18 and 24. The diet should be balanced, with all nutrients balanced proportionally, including carbohydrates. Exercise 30 minutes a day, five days a week. Salt intake affects blood pressure, not blood glucose.

29. D) Phosphorus and calcium
Patients with hypoparathyroidism generally have hypocalcemia and hyperphosphatemia (low calcium and high phosphorus, respectively). The other electrolytes are not affected by hypoparathyroidism.

30. A nurse is caring for a patient diagnosed with hyperthyroidism. Which medication should the nurse be prepared to administer to treat the patient's tachycardia?

    A. Metoprolol
    B. Levothyroxine
    C. Enalapril
    D. Methimazole

31. The nurse is caring for a patient with hypothyroidism. Which nursing diagnosis is appropriate to include in the plan of care?

    A. Decreased fluid volume
    B. Constipation
    C. Bowel incontinence
    D. Anxiety

32. A nurse is caring for a patient with Addison's disease who has the following lab values: sodium 136 mEq/dL, potassium 5.5 mEq/dL, magnesium 2 mEq/dL, calcium 12 mEq/dL. Which medication would the nurse anticipate administering?

    A. Magnesium sulfate
    B. Sodium chloride
    C. Polystyrene sodium
    D. Lactulose

33. A nurse is planning care for a patient with Addison's disease regarding the prescribed cortisone regimen. Which nursing diagnosis should be a priority to include in the teaching plan?

    A. Risk for infection
    B. Nutrition less than body requirements
    C. Risk for injury
    D. Altered skin pigmentation

34. The nurse is caring for patient diagnosed with hypothyroidism. Which nursing diagnosis should the nurse address immediately?

    A. Body image
    B. Alteration in body temperature
    C. Imbalance of caloric intake (more than required)
    D. Depression and withdrawal

35. A nurse is caring for a patient with an alteration in the antidiuretic hormone (ADH). Which diagnostic test should the nurse anticipate will be requested?

    A. Thyroid-stimulating hormone (TSH) test
    B. Abdominal CT scan
    C. Head CT scan
    D. Kidney function test

(See answers next page.)

30. A) Metoprolol

Metoprolol is indicated to treat the sympathetic symptoms associated with hyperthyroidism, including tachycardia, nervousness, and tremors. Levothyroxine is a synthetic version of the thyroid hormone thyroxine. Enalapril is an angiotensin-converting enzyme (ACE) inhibitor used to treat hypertension; methimazole is used to control an overactive thyroid, but does not control tachycardia.

31. B) Constipation

A priority diagnosis for patients with hypothyroidism is constipation due to a generalized slowing down of all body functions, including a weakening of the large and small bowel muscle contractions needed for evacuation. Bowel incontinence and anxiety could be present in hyperthyroidism. Decreased fluid volume is not part of hypothyroidism.

32. C) Polystyrene sodium

The patient has hyperkalemia associated with Addison's disease. The correct medication for the hyperkalemia is polystyrene sodium, a potassium binder. The other labs are within normal limits, so no treatment is indicated.

33. A) Risk for infection

A patient with Addison's disease who is prescribed corticosteroids has a higher risk for developing an infection due to the medications' actions to decrease the inflammation process, decrease the activity of the immune system, and mask signs of potential infections such as fever. Patients with Addison's disease tend to be thin and have skin discoloration, and are at risk for injury during Addisonian crisis; however, those diagnoses are not related to the intake of corticosteroids and are not a priority.

34. D) Depression and withdrawal

Patients with hypothyroidism often suffer from depression, isolation, and withdrawal from others, which increase the risk for suicide. There may be an altered body image due to weight gain; this issue, along with alteration in temperature and caloric imbalances, needs to be addressed but not as a priority.

35. C) Head CT scan

Patients with antidiuretic hormone alteration have an issue with the pituitary gland not secreting adequate ADH. A head CT is indicated to diagnose the disease by visualizing the pituitary gland's size, location, and shape. A TSH test is used in thyroid diagnostics, and an abdominal CT is used to diagnose adrenal issues. A kidney function test is used to diagnose renal disease.

36. The nurse is planning an in-service about health-promotion activities for patients with Cushing's syndrome. Which information should the nurse include in the teaching plan?

    A. Increase the intake of potassium.
    B. Increase the intake of sodium.
    C. Increase the intake of carbohydrates.
    D. Increase weight-bearing exercises.

(See answers next page.)

36. A) Increase the intake of potassium.
Patients with Cushing's syndrome develop hypokalemia, hypernatremia, hyperglycemia, and osteoporosis. Encouraging a patient to increase potassium intake is essential to include in the teaching plan. Increasing intake of sodium or carbohydrates will make the condition worse. Weight-bearing exercises can increase the risk of fractures secondary to osteoporosis.

Immune System

1. Which assessment finding would be a sign of systemic lupus erythematosus (SLE)?

   A. Occurrence of tremors in the patient's hands at rest
   B. Noted contractures to the patient's fingers
   C. Development of a butterfly-shaped rash on the patient's face
   D. Slurred speech and ptosis of the patient's right eye

2. The nurse is working with a physical therapist to create a care plan for a patient with rheumatoid arthritis. What is a priority nursing focus to help promote self-care practices in a patient with this condition?

   A. Ensure that the patient has adequate pain management.
   B. Assist the patient in finding adaptive tools to help with dressing and bathing.
   C. Work with a physical therapist to help prevent joint deformity.
   D. Provide emotional support for the patient.

3. The nurse is evaluating a patient's understanding of celiac disease and diet. Which statement best represents the patient's understanding of dietary restrictions for celiac disease?

   A. "It is important to restrict foods high in potassium."
   B. "I will be unable to eat foods that contain gluten."
   C. "I will need to limit eating foods high in vitamin K."
   D. "I will need to read labels to find food low in sodium."

4. A patient with a history of type 1 diabetes mellitus is started on insulin via an insulin pump. Which of the following types of insulin are administered in an insulin pump for premeal bolus?

   A. Combined/mixed insulin
   B. Long-acting insulin
   C. Rapid-acting insulin
   D. Intermediate-acting insulin

5. A patient recently diagnosed with psoriasis asks the nurse about potential triggers for this condition. How should the nurse respond?

   A. "Psoriasis may be trigged by a recent bacterial or viral infection."
   B. "Psoriasis is linked to vitamin B12 deficiency."
   C. "There are no known triggers for psoriasis symptoms."
   D. "Psoriasis is commonly triggered by weight loss."

(See answers next page.)

1. C) Development of a butterfly-shaped rash on the patient's face

SLE typically presents as an erythematous facial rash in the shape of a butterfly. Other signs include increased temperature, increased respiration rate, increased blood pressure, fatigue, depression, withdrawal, headache, vertigo, and insomnia. Tremors in the hands is a sign of Parkinson's disease. Noted contractures of the fingers occur in rheumatoid arthritis. Slurred speech and ptosis are associated with cerebral vascular accidents (CVA).

2. A) Ensure that the patient has adequate pain management.

The patient will be unable to engage in self-care practices if pain control is not achieved. A priority nursing focus is to ensure that the patient is achieving pain relief. Adaptive tools are suggested in advanced stages of the disease. Physical therapy can help to prevent joint deformity. However, physical therapy is more successful with pain management. Although emotional support is important, pain management will lead to better patient coping and self-care practices.

3. B) "I will be unable to eat foods that contain gluten."

Patients with celiac disease must avoid foods that contain gluten. Exposure to gluten can cause inflammation and increased permeability in the bowel, which leads to intestinal damage. Patients with renal pathologies should avoid foods high in potassium. Patients taking anticoagulant therapy should avoid foods high in vitamin K. Patients with hypertension and heart failure should avoid foods high in sodium.

4. C) Rapid-acting insulin

Even though insulin pumps administer a basal rate of insulin, they use rapid- or short-acting insulin to control blood glucose levels prior to eating. Intermediate and intermediate/short-acting combination insulins are not administered intravenously or via insulin pumps. Long-acting insulin (basal insulin) may be administered via insulin pump, but it is not used as a premeal bolus.

5. A) "Psoriasis may be trigged by a recent bacterial or viral infection."

Psoriasis may be triggered by recent viral or bacterial infections, stress, smoking, weight gain, and vitamin D deficiency. Vitamin B12 does not influence this condition. Having one or both parents with the condition also increases the risk of acquiring it.

6. A 20-year-old patient with type 1 diabetes mellitus is experiencing hypoglycemia during exercise. What should the nurse recommend to ensure patient safety?

   A. "It may be helpful to take your insulin before you start exercising."
   B. "It is helpful to monitor your blood glucose levels after you have finished exercising."
   C. "You should eat foods that have a high glycemic index prior to exercising."
   D. "You should have a carbohydrate-rich snack and exercise 1 hour after eating."

7. A patient with psoriasis is using calcipotriene, a vitamin D analogue. What would be an expected outcome of this pharmacological therapy on affected areas?

   A. The patient has decreased plaque buildup.
   B. The patient has noted smoothness and decreased inflammation.
   C. The patient has decreased pruritus.
   D. The patient has noted thinning of the skin.

8. A 21-year-old female patient is taking romiplostim to treat immune thrombocytopenic purpura (ITP). Which of the following nursing diagnoses applies to this patient?

   A. At risk for deep vein thrombosis related to increased platelet production
   B. At risk for impaired oxygenation related to dyspnea
   C. Impaired skin integrity related to injection site
   D. Potential for confusion due to anemia

9. A patient with HIV is taking anti-retroviral medication therapy. The patient's viral load is now undetectable. What should the nurse teach the patient regarding health promotion and the safety of others?

   A. The patient is now free from the HIV infection and can stop medication therapy.
   B. The patient can now donate blood and share toothbrushes and razors with others.
   C. The patient should understand that they still need to engage in safe-sex practices.
   D. The patient will restart antiretroviral medication therapy if the viral load starts to increase.

10. The nurse evaluates the patient's response to a blood transfusion. The patient has signs of acute renal failure. What type of hypersensitivity reaction has occurred?

    A. Type I hypersensitivity reaction
    B. Type II hypersensitivity reaction
    C. Type III hypersensitivity reaction
    D. Type IV hypersensitivity reaction

(See answers next page.)

6. D) "You should have a carbohydrate-rich snack and exercise 1 hour after eating."

Hypoglycemia may occur during exercise in patients with type 1 diabetes mellitus. The nurse should educate the patient to schedule exercise 1 hour after eating and/or ensure that the patient has a carbohydrate-rich snack (10–15 g) before exercising. The client should monitor the blood glucose before and after exercise, but the snack is the most important factor for safety. High carbohydrates will provide more support than foods with a high glycemic index. The patient will need to eat before, not after exercise.

7. B) The patient has noted smoothness and decreased inflammation.

Vitamin D analogues (e.g., calcipotriene) slow skin cell growth. This results in decreased inflammation and smoother skin. Calcineurin inhibitors (e.g., tacrolimus) reduce plaque buildup. Decreased pruritus is a result of topical corticosteroid use. Noted thinning of the skin results from overuse of topical corticosteroids.

8. A) At risk for deep vein thrombosis related to increased platelet production

Romiplostim is a medication that stimulates the bone marrow to produce more platelets. Patients taking this medication are at risk for deep vein thrombosis and clotting. The nurse must evaluate treatment and ensure that there are not any clinical signs of this complication. The patient is not at impaired risk for oxygenation due to dyspnea in this condition. Romiplostim is administered subcutaneously and has risks similar to other subcutaneous medications, but it does not have a higher risk of impairing skin integrity. Confusion in ITP is due to the rare complication of intracranial bleeding.

9. C) The patient should understand that they still need to engage in safe-sex practices.

Even though the patient has an undetectable viral load, it doesn't mean that HIV isn't present in the body. The patient will need to continue medication therapy and engage in safe sexual practices. It is not recommended that the patient stop medication therapy. In order to prevent transmission of the virus, the patient should not donate blood or share razors, toothbrushes, or other personal items. Antiretroviral medications are not stopped and restarted; it is recommended that patients continue with the therapy.

10. B) Type II hypersensitivity reaction

A type II hypersensitivity reaction (cytotoxic and cytolytic reaction) can occur after a blood transfusion. Hemolytic transfusion reactions occur when a recipient receives ABO-incompatible blood. Renal failure can result from hemoglobinuria. A type I hypersensitivity reaction is an anaphylactic reaction. A type III hypersensitivity reaction is an immune-complex reaction, and a type IV hypersensitivity reaction is a delayed hypersensitivity reaction.

11. A nurse refuses to care for a patient with HIV because the nurse is concerned about personal safety. Which of the following statements best represents the nurse's duty to treat this patient?

    A. The nurse is ethically bound to care for patients who may have infectious blood or other body fluids.

    B. The nurse may refuse patient care if it comes into conflict with the nurse's religious beliefs.

    C. If there is a greater potential for harm to the nurse than the patient, it is appropriate for the nurse to refuse care.

    D. The nurse may refuse care if the nurse is concerned that the nurse may be at risk for infection.

(See answers next page.)

11. A) The nurse is ethically bound to care for patients who may have infectious blood or other body fluids.

Every day, nurses have contact with patients who may have infectious blood or body fluids. Infection precautions are instituted to protect the nurse from transmission. Nurses would have to notify the nurse manager in advance if they had any deeply held religious convictions that might prevent them from giving patient care. In this case, it would be difficult for the nurse to argue that they were at a greater risk by caring for this patient unless the nurse was immunosuppressed. If a nurse's concern is focused on risk of infection, that person may need to reconsider the commitment to the nursing profession.

Urinary System

1. The nurse is caring for a patient with acute kidney injury (AKI). Which nursing diagnoses should be included in the plan of care?

   A. Fluid imbalance: overload
   B. Risk for decreased cardiac output
   C. Risk for impaired skin integrity
   D. Ineffective tissue perfusion

2. The nurse is teaching a patient with end-stage renal failure with hyperphosphatemia. Which information about phosphorus binders is essential to include in the teaching plan?

   A. Take the medication at night.
   B. Take the medication with meals.
   C. Take the medication on an empty stomach.
   D. Take the medication first thing in the morning.

3. The nurse is teaching a recently graduated nurse about using the arteriovenous fistula for hemodialysis. What information should the nurse include in the teaching plan?

   A. Do not auscultate the fistula.
   B. Take the pulse by feeling the bruit in the fistula.
   C. Take the blood pressure on the side opposite the fistula.
   D. Use the fistula to withdraw blood.

4. The nurse is caring for a patient with acute kidney injury (AKI). For which of the following electrolyte imbalances should the nurse anticipate the administration of polystyrene sulfonate?

   A. Sodium of 134 mEq/dL
   B. Potassium of 5.5 mEq/dL
   C. Calcium of 12 mEq/dL
   D. Magnesium of 2.5 mEq/dL

5. The nurse is teaching a patient with end-stage kidney disease who is scheduled for the creation of a fistula. What should the nurse teach the patient about the fistula creation?

   A. During surgery, a vein and an artery will be joined together.
   B. The patient won't be able to move the involved arm for a week.
   C. One needle will be injected in the venous portion of the fistula.
   D. The fistula will be ready to use immediately.

1. A) Fluid imbalance: overload
Patients with AKI have a fluid overload due to the kidneys' inability to eliminate urine effectively. Risk for decreased cardiac output applies to patients with a decreased circulatory volume. Ineffective tissue perfusion applies to O_2 alteration, not to AKI. Risk for impaired skin integrity does not apply in this scenario.

2. B) Take the medication with meals.
Phosphorus binders work by attaching to the phosphorus in food in an effort to eliminate the excess mineral. They work best if given with food, so instructions to take the medication at night, on an empty stomach, or first thing in the morning are not appropriate.

3. C) Take the blood pressure on the side opposite the fistula.
Vital signs should be taken in a site opposite to the fistula, using the opposite arm. The nurse can and should auscultate the fistula to ensure patency. A fistula for dialysis should not be used for purposes other than for hemodialysis, due to its fragility. Drawing blood is not allowed because it could potentially damage the fistula.

4. B) Potassium of 5.5 mEq/dL
Polystyrene sulfonate is the medication of choice to treat hyperkalemia. It is in the class of potassium removal agents, binding potassium and removing it via the intestines.

5. A) During surgery, a vein and an artery will be joined together.
The creation of a fistula attaches a vein to an artery, providing vascular access for frequent hemodialysis treatments. The patient will be able to move the arm after surgery; however, the fistula will have to "mature" before it can be used in dialysis (usually in 4–8 weeks). Two needles will be inserted during each dialysis session to facilitate filtration by the dialysis machine.

6. A nurse is caring for a patient who is in the diuretic phase of acute kidney injury (AKI). For which complication should the nurse monitor during this phase?

   A. Decreased potassium levels

   B. Decreased urinary output

   C. Dehydration

   D. Fluid overload

7. The nurse is caring for a patient who underwent lithotripsy 24 hours ago. Which nurse observation requires further follow-up?

   A. The patient's urine became cloudy.

   B. The patient's fluid intake was 2 L/d.

   C. The nurse observes sand-like particles in the urine.

   D. The patient reports pink-tinged urine sometime during the day.

8. The nurse is caring for a patient with urolithiasis. How much fluid should the nurse recommend the patient drink each day?

   A. 1,700 mL

   B. 1,500 mL

   C. 2,000 mL

   D. 500 mL

9. The nurse is caring for a patient with a urinary disorder who is waiting for a diagnostic ultrasound. The patient was scheduled to have the ultrasound done hours ago. Which of the following actions represents advocacy by the nurse?

   A. Educate the patient about the need for the ultrasound.

   B. Call the radiology department and explain the need to complete the procedure quickly.

   C. Contact the physician for an alternative procedure.

   D. Write an incident report about the length of the delay.

10. The nurse is caring for a patient with chronic kidney disease who speaks only Spanish. The patient's physician speaks only English and needs to give recommendations for specific drinks that would be helpful for the patient. The nurse is fluent in both languages. In which situation is the nurse acting as an advocate for the patient?

    A. The nurse translates the physician's recommendations for the patient.

    B. The nurse contacts the supervisor to report the situation and ask for a translator.

    C. The nurse writes an incident report due to the language barrier.

    D. The nurse contacts the quality-assurance department to report the situation.

(*See answers next page.*)

6. C) Dehydration

During the diuretic phase of AKI, patients will experience increased urinary output, which increases their risk for dehydration. Fluid overload, decreased potassium level, and decreased urinary output are not applicable during the diuretic phase of AKI.

7. A) The patient's urine became cloudy.

During a lithotripsy, sound waves are used to break up stones in the bladder, kidney, or ureter. The nurse needs to report cloudy urine after a lithotripsy because this can be a sign of an infection. Drinking 2 L of fluids daily is recommended to prevent infection and to ensure hydration. After a lithotripsy, having sand-like particles and/or pink-tinged urine is normal.

8. C) 2,000 mL

Urolithiasis occurs when stones form in the bladder, kidney, or urinary tract, causing pain and bleeding. The nurse should recommend a total intake of 2,000 mL a day to continue to flush the urinary tract system adequately; lesser amounts are considered inadequate for urolithiasis.

9. B) Call the radiology department and explain the need to complete the procedure quickly.

By calling the radiology department, the nurse is acting on behalf of the patient to complete the needed procedure in a timely manner. Educating the patient about the procedure should have already occurred, as the patient is waiting for the procedure. Contacting the physician for an alternative procedure or writing an incident report does not represent advocacy but is more reactionary in response.

10. A) The nurse translates the physician's recommendations for the patient.

Helping with the translation demonstrates that the nurse is acting on behalf of the patient, especially because the nurse can help the patient understand the medical need in their native language. The other actions do not demonstrate the role of advocacy. Because the nurse speaks Spanish, there is no need for a translator, nor is it necessary to write an incident report or notify the quality-assurance department.

11. The nurse is conducting an educational seminar for a group of nurses about urinary tract infections (UTIs) in older men. Which of the following statements by the seminar attendees demonstrates that the teaching has been effective?

    A. The incidence of UTIs in older men is equal to the incidence of UTIs in women in the same age group.
    B. It is difficult to determine the incidence of UTIs in older men because men don't report UTIs.
    C. Older men are more prone to UTIs than women are.
    D. Older men are less prone to UTIs but experience more severe symptoms than women of the same age.

12. The charge nurse is observing a new graduate caring for a patient who has just undergone lithotripsy. Which action requires intervention from the charge nurse?

    A. The nurse administers a 1,000-mL bolus of 0.9% saline following the procedure.
    B. The nurse monitors the patient's fluid volume status after the procedure.
    C. The nurse inserts a urinary catheter after the procedure.
    D. The nurse strains the patient's urine after the procedure.

13. The nurse is caring for a patient with a renal disorder secondary to use of a nephrotoxic drug. What should the nurse do to determine whether there is a change in the patient's renal function?

    A. Observe for changes in the skin color.
    B. Observe the amount of the urinary output.
    C. Assess for an abdominal bruit.
    D. Measure temperature status.

14. A patient with chronic kidney disease (CKD) develops deep and labored breathing. The nurse determines that the cause of this response is:

    A. An increase in the serum bicarbonate (HCO_3).
    B. An increase in the serum carbon dioxide (CO_2).
    C. An increase in the serum pH.
    D. A decrease in the serum CO_2.

15. A patient with a glomerular filtration rate (GFR) less than 15 mL/hr has been put on fluid restrictions. Which assessment finding indicates that the patient did not follow the fluid restrictions?

    A. Crackles and dyspnea at rest
    B. Decreased weight
    C. Blood pressure of 90/40 mmHg
    D. Capillary refill longer than 5 seconds

(See answers next page.)

11. A) The incidence of UTIs in older men is equal to the incidence of UTIs in women in the same age group.

The incidence of UTIs in older men is equal to the incidence of UTIs in women in the same age group. Men report UTIs at the same rate as women do. Older men are equally prone to UTIs, but their symptoms are not as severe as women's of the same age.

12. C) The nurse inserts a urinary catheter after the procedure.

Patients are encouraged to void after undergoing lithotripsy; therefore, placement of a urinary catheter is not an expected action. Patients with urinary issues may develop a fluid imbalance, so a bolus of intravenous (IV) fluids may be ordered. Straining the urine is an appropriate intervention after a lithotripsy to identify fragments of stones that were broken up by the procedure.

13. B) Observe the amount of the urinary output.

Observing the urinary output is the best safety intervention to determine positive changes in renal function. Measuring the patient's temperature, observing for skin color changes, or assessing for an abdominal bruit are not interventions that directly determine changes in the renal function.

14. B) An increase in the serum carbon dioxide (CO_2).

Kussmaul respirations are often seen in patients with CKD and metabolic acidosis. The body tries to compensate for the state of acidosis by developing deep and labored breathing to eliminate the CO_2. An increase in the serum bicarbonate and an increase in the pH will cause an alkalotic state, not an acidotic state. Excited breathing, not labored breathing, can cause a decrease in serum CO_2.

15. A) Crackles and dyspnea at rest

Patients with a GFR less than 15 mL/hr are in end-stage renal disease. They are prone to fluid overload, so it is imperative to restrict fluids. Crackles and dyspnea at rest indicate pulmonary edema. Decreased weight, decreased blood pressure, and a capillary refill longer than 5 seconds indicate fluid deficit, not excess.

16. The nurse is caring for a group of patients with renal disorders. To safely delegate nursing tasks, which action can the nurse delegate to unlicensed assistive personnel (UAP)?

    A. Weigh a patient before dialysis.
    B. Check the patency of an arteriovenous fistula.
    C. Assess the patient's lungs for crackles.
    D. Educate the patient about a low-sodium diet.

17. The nurse is reviewing the labs of a patient with chronic renal failure. The glomerular filtration rate (GFR) is 60 mL/min/1.73 m². The nurse understands that the patient's chronic kidney disease is at what stage?

    A. Stage 1
    B. Stage 2
    C. Stage 3
    D. Stage 4

18. A nurse is admitting a patient with nephrotic syndrome. Which clinical finding indicates effectiveness of the therapy?

    A. Decreased weight
    B. Increased edema
    C. Increased blood pressure
    D. Decreased urine output

19. Which of the following patients has the greatest risk for developing end-stage kidney disease (ESKD)?

    A. A patient with polycystic kidney disease
    B. A patient with urolithiasis
    C. A patient with poorly controlled diabetes
    D. A patient with a history of acute renal failure

20. A patient with acute kidney injury has a tall T wave on the EKG that was not noted on the previous shift. Which action should be the priority for the nurse?

    A. Document the finding.
    B. Contact the rapid respond team.
    C. Check the patient's blood urea nitrogen (BUN) and creatinine levels.
    D. Review the patient's most recent serum potassium levels.

21. The nurse is teaching a patient with end-stage kidney disease (ESKD) about disease management. Which statement by the patient indicates that the teaching was effective?

    A. "The amount of liquid I can drink is based on my daily urinary output."
    B. "Erythropoietin will help my immune system."
    C. "I will have no sodium restriction on my diet."
    D. "My kidney function will improve if I take my medications consistently."

(See answers next page.)

16. A) Weigh a patient before dialysis.

A nurse should safely delegate tasks to UAPs according to their training, competency, and standards. Weighing a patient is an appropriate task to delegate. Assessing and teaching tasks are nursing responsibilities requiring a registered nursing license, as is checking the patency of an arteriovenous fistula.

17. B) Stage 2

Patients with chronic renal failure are classified in five stages based on the GFR. Stage 1 is GFR >90 mL/min; Stage 2 is 60 to 89 mL/min; Stage 3 is 30 to 59 mL/min; Stage 4 is 15 to 29 mL/min; Stage 5 is less than 15 mL/min. This patient is in Stage 2.

18. A) Decreased weight

Patients with nephrotic syndrome manifest edema secondary to protein loss in the urine, which creates excess fluid volume. A weight loss indicates improvement in the condition. Increased edema and decreased urinary output indicate disease. Increased blood pressure is not a sign of improvement.

19. C) A patient with poorly controlled diabetes

Diabetes is the number one cause of renal failure in the United States. Uncontrolled diabetes leads to an increased risk for chronic renal failure. A history of acute renal failure is not a high risk factor. Patients with urolithiasis have an increased risk for acute kidney injury (AKI), not diabetes. Patients with polycystic kidney disease are not at high risk for ESKD.

20. D) Review the patient's most recent serum potassium levels.

Patients with acute kidney failure develop hyperkalemia secondary to abnormal kidney function, showing on the EKG as tall T waves. The nurse should check the patient's most recent potassium level. BUN and creatinine levels are not reflected on the EKG. This is not a life-threatening situation requiring a call to the rapid response team; only documenting the finding is a failure to report an abnormality.

21. A) "The amount of liquid I can drink is based on my daily urinary output."

The patient with ESKD has a risk for fluid overload due to the reduced filtration rate of the kidneys. The amount of fluid intake replacement should be calculated based on the daily urinary output. Erythropoietin helps to prevent anemia. Sodium restriction is implemented to prevent fluid retention. In ESKD, the damage is irreversible regardless of the patient's compliance with medications.

22. The nurse is caring for a patient with a renal disorder. The nurse understands that the best indicator of fluid gain or loss is:

    A. Heart rate.
    B. Presence of edema.
    C. Body weight.
    D. Increased blood pressure.

23. The nurse is caring for a mentally competent patient with end-stage renal failure and diabetes. The patient has been consuming a high-calorie, high-sodium diet despite having been informed of the potential consequences of eating this type of diet. What action by the nurse illustrate the nurse's role as a patient advocate?

    A. Ask the family to remove all salt and sugary products from the house.
    B. Advise the patient that this behavior is an end-of-life action.
    C. Accept the patient's choice and do not seek further intervention.
    D. Report the behavior to the primary care provider, because the patient is not compliant with care.

24. While caring for a patient with urolithiasis, the nurse notes an increase in the patient's weight compared with the previous day. Which nursing diagnosis does this finding suggest?

    A. Fluid imbalance: overload
    B. Cardiac output: increased
    C. Imbalanced caloric intake: more than body requirements
    D. Sedentary lifestyle

25. A nurse is teaching a female patient undergoing a bladder training program as treatment for urinary incontinence. Which of the following techniques should the nurse include in the teaching plan?

    A. Take a warm sitz bath three times a day.
    B. Use the smallest catheter for self-catheterization.
    C. Perform Kegel exercises multiple times during the day.
    D. Take anticholinergics three times a day.

26. The nurse is teaching a female patient with frequent urinary tract infections. Which instruction should the nurse include in the teaching plan?

    A. Clean the perineal area from back to front.
    B. Drink 2 L of fluids daily.
    C. Void three times a day.
    D. Refrain from voiding after sex.

(See answers next page.)

22. C) Body weight.

To assess a patient's hydration status, the initial indicator of fluid loss or gain is the body weight. An increased heart rate, presence of edema, and increased blood pressure are all symptoms of increased fluid retention, but not the best indicators.

23. C) Accept the patient's choice and do not seek further intervention.

By accepting the patient's choice, the nurse is fulfilling the role of a patient's advocate. An end-stage patient has the right to eat high-calorie food even though others may believe this is wrong. Asking the family to remove the high-calorie food is against patient's wishes and not realistic. Advising the patient about their behavior does not illustrate the advocacy role, nor does reporting the patient to the healthcare provider.

24. A) Fluid imbalance: overload

Patients with urolithiasis can retain fluids due to the obstruction in the lower urinary system, which could lead to an acute kidney infection (AKI). Fluid imbalance overload is an appropriate nursing diagnosis. There may be a decrease in cardiac output in AKI, not an increase, as fluids may be retained. An imbalance in nutrition or a sedentary lifestyle are not applicable nursing diagnoses for AKI.

25. C) Perform Kegel exercises multiple times during the day.

Kegel exercises are used to increase the bladder sphincter tone. They should be done multiple times during the day. Sitz baths do not help with bladder retraining and self-catheterization is not indicated in the program. Anticholinergics are contraindicated because of the risk of urinary retention.

26. B) Drink 2 L of fluids daily.

Drinking 2 L of fluids a day will help prevent urinary tract infections. The perineal area should always be cleaned from front to back. Voiding at least every 4 hours and after sex is recommended for preventing urinary tract infections.

27. The patient on a bladder retraining program has 40 mL remaining in the bladder after voiding. Which intervention is appropriate for the nurse to implement?

    A. Insert a straight catheter in the bladder.
    B. Place a Foley catheter immediately.
    C. Document the finding.
    D. Press against the bladder.

28. The nurse is caring for a patient with an ileal conduit. When the nurse evaluates the patient's urinary output, which amount of urine voided will require the nurse to notify the physician?

    A. Less than 80 mL/hr
    B. Less than 100 mL/hr
    C. Less than 150 mL/hr
    D. Less than 30 mL/hr

29. The nurse is assessing a patient who has undergone ileal conduit surgery. When preparing to change the appliance, the nurse understands that:

    A. The appliance should be changed on a daily basis.
    B. The abdominal circumference should be measured prior to application.
    C. The appliance should fit tightly around the stoma to prevent leakage.
    D. The stoma size may change in the upcoming weeks.

30. How is the diagnosis of interstitial cystitis confirmed?

    A. 24-hour urine collection
    B. Urine culture
    C. Bladder biopsy
    D. Abdominal x-ray

31. The nurse is teaching a patient with urinary incontinence how to perform Kegel exercises to assist with bladder retraining. Which statement by the patient indicates a need for additional teaching?

    A. "I will need to sit with my legs slightly apart to do the exercises."
    B. "I need to make sure my bladder is empty before I sit down to do the exercises."
    C. "I will need to hold my pelvic floor muscles tight for 5 to 10 seconds for each repetition."
    D. "I will bear down on my pelvic floor muscles as if I am having a bowel movement."

32. The nurse is teaching a patient with urinary retention who needs to perform self-catheterization. Which statement by the patient indicates the need for further teaching?

    A. "I will perform the procedure every 4 to 6 hours."
    B. "I should apply lubricant to the tip of the catheter before insertion."
    C. "I will wash the catheter with soap and water after use."
    D. "I will use sterile technique each time I perform the procedure."

(See answers next page.)

27. C) Document the finding.
Forty mL of urine remaining in the bladder after voiding is a normal finding. Documenting the finding is the appropriate intervention at this time. No catheter is needed, and pressing the bladder to remove the urine is not recommended because the amount of urine remaining is normal.

28. D) Less than 30 mL/hr
If a patient is voiding less than 30 mL/hr, the nurse must notify the physician because this can be an early sign of acute renal failure. The other volumes are acceptable urinary outputs.

29. D) The stoma size may change in the upcoming weeks.
An ileal conduit is created by making an opening, or stoma, through the abdominal wall and bringing a portion of the ileum through to reroute urine into an external collection pouch. The stoma will shrink and change in appearance during the first 6 weeks; therefore, it should be measured prior to each application change. Appliance devices are changed every 3 to 4 days, depending on the type of device. It is not necessary to measure the abdominal circumference. The appliance should not fit tightly as it may cause stoma damage and pain.

30. C) Bladder biopsy
A bladder biopsy is the diagnostic test used to confirm the presence of interstitial cystitis, which is a chronic bladder issue resulting in feelings of fullness, pain, and pressure in the bladder, along with signs of urinary tract symptoms without an obvious cause. A 24-hour urine collection is used to diagnose problems with the kidney. A urine culture is used to diagnose urinary tract infections. An abdominal x-ray would not show bladder inflammation.

31. D) "I will bear down on my pelvic floor muscles as if I am having a bowel movement."
Kegel exercises are used to strengthen the pelvic floor muscles; share with the patient that it feels like trying to stop urination midstream. Straining as if replicating a bowel movement will increase abdominal pressure, potentially putting the pelvic muscles at risk for injury. Sitting with the legs slightly apart enhances relaxation of these specific muscles. It is highly recommended to do these exercises on an empty bladder so as to not cause unexpected urine leakage. To maximize the strengthening of these muscles, the patient should hold each squeeze steady and tightly for 5 to 10 seconds each.

32. D) "I will use sterile technique each time I perform the procedure."
Self-catheterization is a clean procedure and there is no need to follow sterile technique. Washing the catheter with soap and water, lubricating the tip of the catheter before insertion, and performing the procedure every 4 to 6 hours are appropriate protocols to emphasize when teaching a patient how to self-catheterize.

33. The nurse is caring for a patient with urolithiasis who is reporting excruciating pain. Which nursing intervention will help relieve the pain?

    A. Teach deep-breathing exercises.
    B. Encourage the patient to walk frequently.
    C. Encourage the patient to void every 4 hours.
    D. Limit fluid intake.

34. The nurse is caring for a patient with urinary retention who needs residual urine checks. Which of the following interventions should the nurse implement?

    A. Measure bladder volume immediately after the patient voids.
    B. Document the patient's urinary output per shift.
    C. Establish an every-4-hours schedule to check for residual urine.
    D. Check for residual every time the patient reports the urge to void.

35. A nurse is caring for a patient who is taking an alpha-adrenergic medication for the treatment of hypertension and has urinary incontinence. The patient asks the nurse, "Why am I having incontinence?" The best response by the nurse is:

    A. "This is an adverse reaction that requires medications to decrease overactivity of the bladder."
    B. "The supporting ligaments of your bladder are relaxed. You will need to implement Kegel exercises immediately."
    C. "This is a sign of permanent damage to your bladder sphincter."
    D. "This is a medication side effect that will resolve when you stop taking the medication."

36. The nurse is planning care for a patient with urinary incontinence. Which intervention could help to prevent urinary incontinence?

    A. Use a bedpan frequently.
    B. Administer a diuretic at night.
    C. Increase caffeine consumption.
    D. Empty the bladder every 4 hours.

37. The nurse is planning for removal of a suprapubic catheter from a 90-year-old patient. To safely remove the catheter, the nurse recognizes that the patient's residual urine must be less than what amount?

    A. 140 mL
    B. 150 mL
    C. 100 mL
    D. 200 mL

(See answers next page.)

33. B) Encourage the patient to walk frequently.

Patients with pain secondary to urolithiasis (presence of urinary stones) should be encouraged to walk frequently to decrease the pain. Teaching deep-breathing exercises and encouraging the patient to void every 4 hours will not help with pain. Fluids should be encouraged, not limited, for patients with urolithiasis, to assist in passing the stones.

34. A) Measure bladder volume immediately after the patient voids.

To check for residual urine amounts, the nurse should measure the amount of urine in the bladder immediately after voiding. Any volume less than 50 to 100 mL is normal in older patients, whereas less than 65 mL is desirable for younger patients. Documenting the patient's urinary output does not help to assess residual urine. The patient's residual urine should be assessed after each void, not on a 4-hour schedule, nor when the patient has the urge to void.

35. D) "This is a medication side effect that will resolve when you stop taking the medication."

Alpha-adrenergic drugs are used in patients with both hypertension and urinary retention. Incontinence is a side effect of the alpha-adrenergics. Once the medication is discontinued, the urinary incontinence disappears. Urinary incontinence is not a permanent adverse reaction and there will not be damage to the supporting ligaments or the bladder sphincter.

36. D) Empty the bladder every 4 hours.

A patient with urinary incontinence should be encouraged to empty the bladder every 4 hours. Caffeine increases the risk for incontinence, as caffeine has a diuretic action. Using a bedpan does not help to prevent incontinence. Diuretics will increase urinary output and they are not recommended for administration at night; rather, they are given first thing in the morning.

37. C) 100 mL

Suprapubic catherization is usually discontinued when the volume of residual urine is less than 100 mL. Volumes of 100 mL, 140 mL, or 400 mL are too high to consider removal of the catheter.

38. The nurse is following up the teaching of a patient with chronic cystitis, who is recommended to follow an acid–ash diet. If the teaching was effective, the patient will restrict which beverage?

    A. Milk
    B. Cranberry juice
    C. Plum juice
    D. Prune juice

39. A 76-year-old man complains of difficulty with urination, including difficulty starting to urinate, frequency, and getting up in the middle of the night to urinate. About 500 mL of urine is visible with a bladder scan and catheterization is ordered, but the nurse is unable to complete the procedure due to resistance. What is now indicated as a next step?

    A. Use a smaller-bore catheter.
    B. Apply additional lubricant to the catheter tip.
    C. Place a curved-tipped Coudé catheter.
    D. Gently massage the bladder externally.

40. The nurse is preparing a patient scheduled to undergo a vasectomy. The patient tells the nurse, "I know I signed the consent for this but I still have questions about what choices I have if I would like to have a child in the future." What is the best answer by the nurse?

    A. "You had the chance to ask questions before. Did you ask the doctor about this question specifically?"
    B. "It sounds like you have more questions. Let me call the doctor."
    C. "This is a simple procedure that is reversible."
    D. "Don't worry. You can ask that question in the operating room."

41. The nurse is caring for a male patient who reports burning urination, swollen testicles bilaterally, and a green discharge from the penis. Which of the following diagnosis should the nurse expect to find in this patient?

    A. Chancre
    B. Syphilis
    C. Gonorrhea
    D. Testicular torsion

42. The nurse is teaching a patient with benign prostatic hypertrophy (BPH) about the use of finasteride. Which information should the nurse include in the teaching plan?

    A. Hair loss is an expected side effect.
    B. Erectile dysfunction may occur.
    C. Serious allergic reactions may occur.
    D. Finasteride does not alter the blood test used to detect prostate cancer.

(See answers next page.)

38. A) Milk

The goal in an ash-free diet is to create a more acidic urine to prevent the formation of urinary tract stones. Milk should be avoided because it creates an alkaline ash that increases urinary pH, which in turn increases the risk for cystitis. In addition, beets, kale, and mustard greens are to be avoided. Cranberries, plums, and prunes are allowed in the acid–ash diet, along with high-protein foods such as fish and meats.

39. C) Place a curved-tipped Coudé catheter.

An enlarged prostate is most likely the causative factor in an elderly man who has difficulty voiding. The curved-tipped Coudé catheter is able to go around the enlarged prostate. A smaller-bore catheter may progress, but it can be painful. Massaging the bladder to help with the catheter progression is not helpful, nor is adding lubricant to the catheter tip, as there is an impedance in advancing the catheter.

40. B) "It sounds like you have more questions. Let me call the doctor."

If the patient has questions after signing the consent form, the nurse should contact the doctor to clarify the questions. Asking the patient whether he asked the questions before signing the consent, without offering a solution, is not therapeutic communication and may imply that the patient did not listen effectively. Vasectomy is a procedure that in most cases is permanent; it potentially can be reversed, but there is no guarantee. The patient's doubts should be addressed before sending the patient to surgery.

41. C) Gonorrhea

Gonorrhea is a sexually transmitted disease characterized by painful urination and greenish discharge. If left untreated, it can ascend to the testicles and cause inflammation. Syphilis, which is indicated by a chancre, does not cause discharge from the penis or testicular inflammation. Testicular torsion causes sudden, severe pain in the scrotum and urinary frequency, but not discharge.

42. B) Erectile dysfunction may occur.

Finasteride works by decreasing the amount of a natural body hormone, dihydrotestosterone (DHT), that causes growth of the prostate. This drug may cause sexual dysfunction due to a decrease in DHT. Hair growth is a side effect, and serious allergic reactions are uncommon. Finasteride alters the prostate-specific antigen (PSA) levels, the test used to diagnose prostate cancer.

Musculoskeletal System

1. After being ejected from a car, a 32-year-old male is admitted to the surgical unit with a fracture to the right femur and pelvis. Twenty-six hours later, which early assessment finding would indicate a potential complication?

   A. Tiny, rash-like red spots on the chest area
   B. Decreased erythrocyte sedimentation rate (ESR)
   C. Ongoing swelling to the right leg
   D. Hypothermia

2. After undergoing a total knee replacement, the patient reports pain unrelieved by analgesics. What is the nurse's first priority?

   A. Assess pulses in the affected extremity.
   B. Document the finding.
   C. Administer a pro re nata (PRN) dose of gabapentin (Neurontin).
   D. Call the emergency response team.

3. A patient admitted with crush injuries to the abdomen is at risk for developing which of the following?

   A. Hypokalemia
   B. Rhabdomyolysis
   C. Hypercalcemia
   D. Metabolic alkalosis

4. Which assessment finding would indicate a complication in a patient who has just had a laminectomy?

   A. Pain at the incision site
   B. Urinary incontinence
   C. Decreased appetite
   D. Patient report of feeling groggy and drowsy

5. The nurse is caring for a patient in Buck's traction for a femoral fracture. Which of the following assessment findings should the medical-surgical nurse report to the physician immediately?

   A. The rope is secured in pulley tracts.
   B. The traction weights are on the floor.
   C. The bed is tilted.
   D. Patient reports pain.

1. A) Tiny, rash-like red spots on the chest area

A fat embolism commonly occurs after fractures to the lower-extremity long bones and pelvis; an early sign of this would be a petechial rash. Patients with a fat embolus will have an elevated ESR, not a decreased ESR. Swelling following a long-bone fracture can last several days and would not be a concerning finding at this time. Hyperthermia is an early symptom of a fat embolus, so hypothermia is not a likely finding.

2. A) Assess pulses in the affected extremity.

Paresthesias and pain unrelieved by analgesics or worsening pain are symptoms associated with compartment syndrome. Compartment syndrome can occur within 6 to 8 hours after surgery, resulting in decreased circulation. Therefore, the nurse's first priority is to assess pulses. Although the nurse will also document the finding, this is not the first priority. Administering gabapentin may mask the problem and result in further patient harm. The first priority is to assess the problem, not to call the emergency response team.

3. B) Rhabdomyolysis

Traumatic rhabdomyolysis is a condition that results when skeletal muscle mass is compressed, causing skeletal muscle tissue death. Damaged muscle cells in crush injuries release potassium into the bloodstream, resulting in hyperkalemia, so hypokalemia is not likely to be a risk. Hypocalcemia, not hypercalcemia, may occur due to the release of phosphate in the bloodstream from damaged muscle cells. Patients are at risk for developing metabolic acidosis after crush injuries due to lactic acid buildup.

4. B) Urinary incontinence

Injury to the spinal cord's dura and nerve roots' "cauda equina syndrome" may occur, causing neural tissue damage that can result in bowel/bladder incontinence. Pain at the incision site is an expected finding after a laminectomy. Decreased appetite and feelings of grogginess/drowsiness are expected findings associated with anesthesia.

5. B) The traction weights are on the floor.

Buck's skin traction is used for patients with lower limb fractures, such as femoral fractures. In Buck's traction, the correct amount of weight must be determined per physician orders. The weights should be suspended in the air to ensure traction, so if the nurse finds the weights on the floor or bed, this should be reported to the physician. The ropes should securely fit in the pulley tracts. The bed should be tilted to maintain countertraction. Minimal pain is an expected finding for a patient with femoral fracture in Buck's traction, so the nurse would administer analgesics as ordered.

6. Which of the following diagnoses could result in a C-reactive protein level of 562 mg/L?

    A. Spinal cord injury
    B. Rheumatoid arthritis
    C. Hypertension
    D. Pulmonary embolism

7. The nurse obtains a history from a 33-year-old male admitted with a chief complaint of dark urine and generalized weakness. The patient tells the nurse that his typical daily activities consists of weight training in the morning and high-intensity training in the evening because he is preparing for a fitness competition. Which of the following is the MOST accurate nursing diagnosis based on this information?

    A. Disturbed body image
    B. Impaired physical mobility
    C. Risk for injury
    D. Ineffective sexual pattern

8. Which of the following interventions should the nurse include in the care plan for a patient diagnosed with rhabdomyolysis?

    A. Reduce sodium intake.
    B. Allow patient to lift weights greater than 50 pounds.
    C. Ensure fluid resuscitation.
    D. Increase potassium intake.

9. The nurse witnesses a patient walking to the bathroom suddenly fall and hit their head. The nurse immediately runs to check on the patient and finds them conscious, but complaining of pain. What is the FIRST action the nurse should take?

    A. Apply a pressure dressing to the scalp laceration.
    B. Help the patient up into a wheelchair and back to their bed.
    C. Perform a neurovascular assessment and notify the healthcare provider immediately.
    D. Apply a cervical collar.

10. The nurse is performing an admission assessment on a 32-year-old female patient admitted for right leg pain. The patient denies any medical and surgical history. The patient states that she recently took a 16-hour flight to Greenland. Upon her return, she began having leg cramps. Which of the following labs should the nurse anticipate the physician to order STAT?

    A. D-dimer
    B. Lactic acid
    C. Creatine kinase
    D. Hemoglobin A1C

(See answers next page.)

6. B) Rheumatoid arthritis

C-reactive protein is a biomarker of inflammation. The average level for a normal adult is between 1 mg/L and 3 mg/L. A level above 100 mg/L indicates an inflammatory disorder, such as rheumatoid arthritis. Rheumatoid arthritis is an autoimmune inflammatory disease that affects the joints in the hands and feet. Patients diagnosed with spinal cord injuries, hypertension, or pulmonary embolism would not have C-reactive protein levels above 300 mg/L.

7. C) Risk for injury

The patient is exhibiting signs consistent with rhabdomyolysis, such as dark urine and generalized weakness; therefore, the most accurate nursing diagnosis is risk for injury. The patient is at risk for kidney failure if rhabdomyolysis is left untreated. No objective or subjective data presented indicate that the patient would be at risk for disturbed body image. The patient's age, activity level, and objective symptoms align with a diagnosis of rhabdomyolysis; therefore, ineffective sexual pattern is an assumption and is likely not the most appropriate response.

8. C) Ensure fluid resuscitation.

Restoring extracellular volume early is the number-one treatment priority in patients diagnosed with rhabdomyolysis, so fluid resuscitation is a key intervention. Reducing sodium intake is likely not necessary, and it may delay correction of the problem due to sodium's effect on water. Resuming weight-lifting can exacerbate the problem of muscle cell death. Increasing potassium intake can worsen hyperkalemia, resulting in serious cardiac abnormalities.

9. D) Apply a cervical collar.

Patients who fall and hit the head are at risk for a cervical or skull fracture. Therefore, a cervical collar should be applied immediately after a fall with head injury until imaging is performed. If bleeding is present, a pressure dressing should be applied to the scalp laceration, but this is not a priority action. Moving the patient to chair or bed without stabilizing the cervical spine can result in further patient harm. Although performing a neurovascular assessment may be warranted, this is not the first action because it does not address the patient's safety.

10. A) D-dimer

The patient is exhibiting symptoms consistent with a venous thrombophlebitis, such as cramp-like leg pain after recent long travel. The nurse should anticipate that the physician will order D-dimer levels to be tested. Based on patient data, there is no indication that lactic acid and creatine levels would be useful. Although assessing the patient's hemoglobin A1C might be good for a patient experiencing diabetic neuropathy, this patient has no other medical comorbidities.

11. Which of the following interventions should the nurse include in the care plan for a patient diagnosed with fibromyalgia?

    A. Reassure the patient that with treatment, they will be cured.
    B. Monitor the patient for drug-seeking behaviors.
    C. Encourage the patient to get exercise to promote restorative sleep.
    D. Encourage the patient to introduce more dairy products into their diet.

12. An elderly woman returns to the ED for pain after being casted for a right humerus fracture 2 weeks ago. The patient is admitted to the surgical unit for further evaluation. During the assessment, the nurse notes that the patient's right hand is swollen and discolored. Which of the following actions should the nurse take FIRST?

    A. Administer oxygen.
    B. Elevate the patient's head of bed to improve venous return.
    C. Document the finding.
    D. Assess temperature of the right hand.

13. Which patient response related to osteoporosis indicates a knowledge deficit?

    A. "I will continue weight-bearing exercises."
    B. "I will limit my alcohol intake."
    C. "I will be sure to increase my calcium intake."
    D. "I will replace regular cigarettes with e-cigarettes."

14. A female patient is diagnosed with a comminuted fracture in her right humerus bone. How does the nurse best explain this condition?

    A. A comminuted fracture is seen when there is more than one fracture line, resulting in more than two bone fragments.
    B. A comminuted fracture is seen when a fracture occurs across the entire bone, creating distinct fragments.
    C. A comminuted fracture is seen when the fracture occurs at an approximate 45-degree angle.
    D. A comminuted fracture is seen when multiple pieces of bone are seen at bone ends.

15. The nurse is preparing discharge teaching for a 28-year-old patient going home with a plaster cast on the right foot. Which of the following statements should be included in the discharge teaching?

    A. "Do not touch the cast with your fingers for at least 30 minutes after placement."
    B. "To relieve itching, it is okay to use a warm dryer or tap the cast for relief."
    C. "Keep your foot in a dependent or downward position."
    D. "To relieve itching, it is not okay to insert a thin object underneath the cast."

(See answers next page.)

11. C) Encourage the patient to get exercise to promote restorative sleep.
Fibromyalgia syndrome is characterized by a chronic, nonarticular musculoskeletal pain with unknown cause, occurring often in women ages 30 to 50. Patients who are diagnosed with fibromyalgia complain of extreme fatigue due to sleep deprivation, so patients are encouraged to exercise to promote sleep. There is no cure for fibromyalgia syndrome. Patients with fibromyalgia often have pain and fatigue unrelieved by analgesics; accusing these patients of drug-seeking is an invalid assumption. A possible cause of fibromyalgia is consumption of dairy products, wheat or corn cereal, yeast, caffeine, and citrus.

12. D) Assess temperature of the right hand.
The patient could be experiencing a deep vein thrombosis in the right arm, so the first action of the nurse should be to assess temperature and pulse in the affected extremity. Administering oxygen to the patient is unnecessary and unrelated to the problem. Elevating the head of the bed is helpful, but it will place the affected extremity in a dependent position and the nurse will need to prop the patient's extremity up to improve venous return. The nurse must assess the problem further before documenting it; to do otherwise could delay intervention and result in patient harm.

13. D) "I will replace regular cigarettes with e-cigarettes."
Osteoporosis is a metabolic bone disorder in which the rate of bone resorption exceeds the rate of bone formation, causing a loss of bone mass. Smoking is the most common risk factor for osteoporosis development, so plans to continue to smoke indicate a knowledge deficit. Lifestyle factors associated with the development of osteoporosis are lack of weight-bearing exercise, alcohol use, and inadequate calcium intake.

14. A) A comminuted fracture is seen when there is more than one fracture line, resulting in more than two bone fragments.
A comminuted fracture appears when there is more than one fracture line, resulting in more than two bone fragments. A complete fracture is seen when a fracture occurs across the entire bone, creating distinct fragments. An oblique fracture is seen when the fracture occurs at an approximate 45-degree angle. A burst fracture is seen when multiple pieces of bone are seen at bone ends or in vertebrae.

15. D) "To relieve itching, it is not okay to insert a thin object underneath the cast."
Patients are instructed not to place any foreign objects inside the cast, due to risk for skin breakdown and further injury. A plaster cast should not be touched with fingers, only the palms of hands, for at least 48 to 72 hours after placement while it dries, to avoid indentations that can create pressure points. For itching, it is okay to use cool air, not warm, because warm air can cause more injury to the skin. Patients are instructed to keep an affected extremity elevated to improve venous return and reduce localized swelling.

16. The nurse is preparing discharge teaching for a patient diagnosed with rheumatoid arthritis. The patient is prescribed azathioprine (Imuran). Which of the following medication side effects should the nurse inform the patient of?

    A. Constipation
    B. Increased appetite
    C. Hair loss
    D. Diplopia

17. The patient admitted for a total hip arthroplasty is ready to be discharged. Which of the following actions by the patient would prompt the nurse to intervene immediately?

    A. Ambulating to the bathroom
    B. Lying on their unaffected side
    C. Repositioning the abductor pillow
    D. Bending over to pull up their socks

18. The patient's family asks about the proper use of a cane. Which response is most appropriate?

    A. "Hold the cane in the hand on the affected side, then take a step with the affected leg and bring the cane forward at the same time."
    B. "Hold the cane in the hand on the unaffected side, then take a step with the affected leg and bring the cane forward at the same time."
    C. "Hold the cane in either hand and take a step with the affected leg first."
    D. "Hold the cane in the hand on the unaffected side, then take a step with the unaffected leg and bring the cane forward at the same time."

19. The nurse instructs the client diagnosed with rheumatoid arthritis to avoid which of the following?

    A. Carbohydrates
    B. Exercise
    C. Smoking
    D. Weight loss

20. A nurse is caring for a patient diagnosed with osteoporosis. What should the patient be encouraged to eat more of?

    A. Eggs
    B. Canned foods
    C. Wheat bran
    D. Rhubarb

21. A patient is admitted for a gout flare-up. To reduce flare-ups, the nurse instructs the patient to avoid which foods?

    A. Low-fat dairy products
    B. Wheat
    C. Barley
    D. Liver

(*See answers next page.*)

16. C) Hair loss
Hair loss is a common side effect of azathioprine (Imuran). Diarrhea, not constipation, is another side effect of azathioprine. Diplopia is not a side effect of azathioprine. Loss of appetite, not increased appetite, is a side effect.

17. D) Bending over to pull up their socks
After a total hip arthroplasty, it is very important for patients to move carefully so as not to dislocate the hip. Patients should not bend too far forward at the waist or pull their legs up toward the chest, as this can result in dislocation. Patients who wish to lie on their side must lie on the unaffected side, so this would not prompt immediate attention from the nurse. Recovery is enhanced for patients who are up ambulating as early as possible after surgery. Patients are encouraged to use an abductor pillow to ensure proper hip alignment, so this would likely not prompt the nurse's intervention.

18. B) "Hold the cane in the hand on the unaffected side, then take a step with the affected leg and bring the cane forward at the same time."
Proper cane instructions must be given to the patient to reduce the risk of injury. The patient should hold the cane in the hand on the unaffected side to provide support to the opposite lower limb. A step should be taken with the affected leg and the cane brought forward at the same time. Holding the cane on the affected side or stepping with the unaffecting leg while bringing the cane forward are incorrect. The cane should be held in the hand of the unaffected side only; holding the cane on either side could result in patient injury.

19. C) Smoking
Rheumatoid arthritis is an autoimmune inflammatory disorder that can affect the joint lining, leading to pain, bone erosion, and joint deformity. Smoking can trigger inflammation and increase rheumatoid arthritis flare-ups, so patients should avoid smoking. Patients are encouraged to exercise and eat a well-balanced diet consisting of carbohydrates, fats, and proteins. Patients are encouraged to lose weight to reduce pressure on joints.

20. A) Eggs
Patients with osteoporosis should be instructed to eat foods high in calcium and vitamin D, such as eggs, milk, cheese, and yogurt. Canned and processed foods should be avoided due to the increase salt intake. Wheat bran and rhubarb are high in phytates and oxalates, which prevents the body from absorbing calcium, and should avoided.

21. D) Liver
Organ meats like liver are high in purines, which can increase uric acid levels and lead to gout flare-ups, so they should be avoided. Low-fat dairy products, wheat, and barley are encouraged.

Neurological System

1. A 23-year-old male patient home from college is admitted to the medical–surgical unit for observation. He has severe headaches and generalized muscle aches. Twelve hours after admission, the patient begins vomiting and is overheard shouting at the patient care assistant for turning on the lights to obtain vital signs. The patient care assistant reports the following vital signs: temperature 101.4°F (38.5°C), respiration 20 breaths/min, heart rate 124 beats/min, blood pressure 110/85 mmHg. Which of the following diagnoses would the nurse most likely suspect?

   A. Influenza
   B. Meningococcal disease
   C. Alcohol withdrawal
   D. Acute renal failure

2. The nurse is assigned to a 56-year-old male patient who fell last night while trying to walk to the bathroom. The night nurse reports that the patient has a history of influenza and is now complaining of tingling in both legs. Upon physical assessment, the nurse notes absent deep tendon reflexes bilaterally. The physician orders a lumbar puncture test to assess cerebrospinal fluid (CSF), and the results reveal elevated protein. Which of the following diagnoses would the nurse most likely suspect?

   A. Bacterial meningitis
   B. Diabetes mellitus
   C. Pneumonia
   D. Amyotrophic lateral sclerosis (ALS)

3. Which of the following assessment findings in a supine patient would indicate meningeal inflammation, a medical emergency?

   A. The patient flexes his neck when his knee is extended back.
   B. The patient flexes his feet when his head is tilted toward his chest.
   C. The patient flexes his knees and hips when his head is tilted toward his chest.
   D. The patient flexes his knees and hips when his head is tilted back.

1. B) Meningococcal disease

The patient has tachycardia, fever, muscle aches, irritability, and sensitivity to light. These symptoms are characteristic of meningococcal disease. Meningococcal disease is a condition that affects young adults, especially college students who live in dorms. Although influenza and alcohol withdrawal are possible, they are likely not the cause of the symptoms. Fever with headaches and sensitivity to light should signal meningeal inflammation. Acute renal failure is unrelated to the symptoms presented.

2. D) Amyotrophic lateral sclerosis (ALS)

Elevated protein in CSF along with paresthesias and absent/diminished deep tendon reflexes are indicative of amyotrophic lateral sclerosis, or ALS. ALS (Lou Gehrig's disease) is a neurologic disorder, typically preceded by a respiratory or gastrointestinal infection, that progressively affects motor neuron function leading to ascending paralysis. Although bacterial meningitis is also associated with elevated protein in CSF, this is likely not the cause of the patient's symptoms, as diminished deep tendon reflexes are not a sign of meningitis. Patients with diabetes mellitus may have tingling sensations in both legs, but this is likely not the cause of elevated protein in CSF. Pneumonia is unrelated to the symptoms presented.

3. C) The patient flexes his knees and hips when his head is tilted toward his chest.

A positive sign of meningeal inflammation is Brudzinski's sign, which is a flexing of the hips and knees (an involuntary reaction caused by the inflamed meninges) that occurs when a patient lies supine and his head is tilted to his chest (chin to chest).

4. The nurse is assigned to a 54-year-old male admitted with a chief complaint of nausea and vomiting blood. The patient has a history of a head and neck neoplasm that required laryngectomy and chemoradiation therapy. The night nurse reports that the patient became hypotensive overnight, and 1 L of isotonic fluids was administered. On exam, the patient vomits 300 mL of bright red blood and appears fatigued and pale. Vital signs are blood pressure 101/70 mmHg, temperature 97.5°F (36.4°C), heart rate 117 beats/min, respiration 18 breaths/min, and 91% oxygen saturation on 2 L oxygen via nasal canula. Which of the following actions is most appropriate for the nurse to take?

A. Contact the provider to report the current patient assessment.

B. Insert a nasogastric tube and attach to low-intermittent suction.

C. Submit a blood sample to the lab for type and cross-match.

D. Consult the respiratory therapist for a breathing treatment.

5. While the nurse is assisting a patient out of bed to a standing position to use the urinal, the patient's body suddenly begins to jerk uncontrollably. What is the nurse's immediate priority during the seizure?

A. Insert a tongue blade in the patient's mouth to protect the airway.

B. Observe the duration of the seizure, noting start and end time.

C. Assist the patient to the floor and place a pillow behind his head.

D. Call for help and initiate a rapid response.

6. A patient admitted to the ICU for status epilepticus is transferred to the medical unit. Which of the following lab results would the nurse be concerned about?

A. Hemoglobin 11 g/dL

B. Hematocrit 30% g/dL

C. Phenytoin level 4 mcg/mL

D. White blood cell 7,300/mm

7. A 23-year-old female patient admitted to the ICU for status epilepticus is transferred to the medical–surgical unit. Two hours after transfer, which of the following assessment findings would require immediate notification to the physician?

A. Patient complains of a headache and is sleepy but arousable.

B. Patient has a Glasgow Coma Scale (GCS) score of 15.

C. Patient has a GCS score of 8.

D. Patient has enlarged and inflamed gums.

8. The nurse is caring for a 46-year-old female patient admitted for a hypertensive crisis. The patient care assistant reports that the patient is having difficulty talking and asks the nurse to assess her. On exam, the nurse notices the patient has a left-sided facial droop. What is the most appropriate action for the nurse to take?

A. Activate the rapid response team and prepare the patient for a CT scan.

B. Contact the neurologist for an order to administer a thrombolytic medication.

C. Reassess the patient in 30 minutes.

D. Recommend that the patient be transferred to the neurology step-down unit.

(See answers next page.)

4. A) Contact the provider to report the current patient assessment.

The patient is vomiting bright red blood and has concerning vital signs despite previous interventions, which requires further evaluation. The nurse should first contact the provider to update them on the patient's status and receive subsequent orders. Placing a nasogastric tube and submitting a specimen for type and cross-match are not priority interventions and should not be performed without an order from the provider. The clinical picture does not indicate that a breathing treatment is required.

5. C) Assist the patient to the floor and place a pillow behind his head.

The immediate priority during a witnessed seizure is to protect the patient from injury. The nurse should assist the patient to the floor to protect him from falling and head trauma. Never place anything in the patient's mouth or restrain the patient, because this is likely to result in tooth damage or further injury. After they are placed in a position that protects them from injury, it is recommended to turn patients to one side to protect the airway. The next action would be to observe the duration of the seizure, but this does not supersede patient safety. Although calling for help is warranted, this action is not considered an immediate intervention.

6. C) Phenytoin level 4 mcg/mL

A normal phenytoin level is 10 to 20 mcg/mL; therefore, a phenytoin level of 4 mcg/mL means the drug level is not within therapeutic range. Leukopenia is a side effect of phenytoin; however, the patient's white blood cell count is within normal range. The hemoglobin and hematocrit results are also within normal ranges.

7. C) Patient has a GCS score of 8.

A GCS score of 8 or lower warrants intubation to protect the patient's airway, so it should be reported to the physician immediately. In the postictal phase, it is expected for the patient to be tired and she may also have a headache. A GCS score of 15 indicates mild dysfunction; however, a score of 8 or lower is a concern. Gingival hyperplasia is a side effect of phenytoin, which is an anticonvulsant.

8. A) Activate the rapid response team and prepare the patient for a CT scan.

The most appropriate action is to activate a rapid response and begin preparing the patient for a CT scan, because the patient is demonstrating signs of a stroke. Contacting the neurologist for a thrombolytic prior to knowing the type of stroke the patient is having is not recommended, because if the patient has a hemorrhagic stroke a thrombolytic would increase bleeding. Interventions after a brain infarct are time sensitive, so waiting 30 minutes before intervening can result in more patient harm. Recommending a transfer to the neuro step-down unit is not the most appropriate action at this time because it is essential to initiate a CT scan within 25 minutes of symptom presentation.

9. A 76-year-old male patient is transferred to the medical–surgical unit after having a thrombotic stroke. The physician orders a regular diet for the patient. Shortly after, a dietary representative delivers the patient's tray to the bedside. Which of the following actions by the nurse is most appropriate?

   A. Remove the tray from the bedside and put the patient on nothing-by-mouth (NPO) status until the physician orders a thickening agent.
   B. Contact the neurologist for an order to implement aspiration precautions.
   C. Remove the tray from the bedside and contact the speech therapist for a dysphagia screening.
   D. Delegate feeding to the patient care assistant and implement aspiration precautions.

10. A female patient is prescribed phenytoin (Dilantin) 100 mg three times a day for a seizure disorder. Which of the following statements made by the patient would indicate a knowledge deficit?

   A. "I can switch between generic phenytoin and brand-name Dilantin."
   B. "I will notify the physician prior to stopping this medication."
   C. "I will regularly schedule dental appointments."
   D. "I will stop taking my birth control pills and use a condom/diaphragm with spermicides instead."

11. A 72-year-old female patient is transferred to the medical unit after a thrombotic stroke. During the assessment, the nurse notices that the patient has mild nystagmus. Which of the following cranial nerves is affected?

   A. Cranial nerve I
   B. Cranial nerve X
   C. Cranial nerve IX
   D. Cranial nerve III

12. A patient is admitted to the medical–surgical unit for cocaine abuse. During hourly rounding, the nurse notices that the patient begins jerking uncontrollably and this episode lasts longer than 5 minutes. After ensuring patient safety, the nurse calls a rapid response. The first line of treatment to abort the seizure is:

   A. Oral carbamazepine (Tegretol).
   B. Intravenous lorazepam (Ativan).
   C. Intramuscular valproic acid (Depakene).
   D. Intravenous phenobarbital.

(See answers next page.)

9. C) Remove the tray from the bedside and contact the speech therapist for a dysphagia screening.
Difficulty with swallowing (dysphagia) happens after a stroke because the brain does not activate muscle reflexes at the back of the throat quickly enough, placing the patient at risk for aspiration. After a stroke, patients must be evaluated for dysphagia before they eat; thus, ordering a thickening agent is not recommended until a dysphagia screening is completed. After the patient has been screened for dysphagia and cleared to eat, aspiration precautions should be implemented. Although a nurse may delegate feeding to the patient care assistant, this is likely not the most appropriate action until after the patient has been cleared to eat by a speech therapist.

10. A) "I can switch between generic phenytoin and brand-name Dilantin."
The patient should be maintained on either the generic or brand-name version of the medication. Switching between the two options can cause alterations in drug levels and places the patient at risk for seizures. It is recommended that the patient notify the physician prior to stopping this medication. Gingival hyperplasia is a side effect of phenytoin, so patients are encouraged to visit their dentist regularly and practice good dental hygiene. Phenytoin can lessen the effectiveness of birth control pills, so it is recommended for patients to use additional contraceptive alternatives.

11. D) Cranial nerve III
Cranial nerves III, IV, and VI (oculomotor, trochlear, and abducens) are responsible for extraocular movements; when they are affected, nystagmus can result. Cranial nerve I (olfactory) is responsible for smell. Cranial nerves IX and X (glossopharyngeal and vagus) are responsible for oral motor functions, such as swallowing.

12. B) Intravenous lorazepam (Ativan).
Intravenous benzodiazepines are the preferred first-line agents for patients experiencing status epilepticus. Carbamazepine and valproic acid are prescribed for tonic–clonic seizures. Phenobarbital is a second- or third-line drug for status epilepticus.

13. The nurse is conducting discharge teaching to a patient following an embolic stroke. The patient has a history of hypertension and tobacco abuse. During the teaching, the patient asks, "If I stop smoking, eat healthy, and start exercising, would I still have to take all these medications?" Which response would be most appropriate for the nurse to make?

    A. "No, you could stop taking the medications because making those changes would help to reduce the risk factors for developing another stroke."
    B. "No, you would no longer have to take these medications, but you would need to start checking your blood pressure daily."
    C. "I don't know; would you like for me to contact your physician?"
    D. "Those changes would help to reduce the risk factors for developing another stroke; however, speak with your physician before you stop taking your medications."

14. The nurse is caring for a patient who had a cerebrovascular injury and has residual weakness. The patient states, "I will never be the same!" Which statement made by the nurse is most therapeutic?

    A. "With rehabilitation, you will return back to baseline so don't worry yourself."
    B. "It's normal to feel this way after a stroke. The goal of physical therapy is to help you get as close to your normal self as possible."
    C. "Would you like to speak with a psychologist about your concerns?"
    D. "Everything is going to be fine. You should focus on rehabilitation."

15. The nurse is assigned to a 54-year-old male admitted with a chief complaint of severe migraine. The patient informs the nurse that 3 weeks ago, he injured his spinal cord at levels T4 to T6. While examining the patient, the nurse notes that the bedside telemetry monitor shows multiple premature ventricular contractions and the patient's skin is flushed. The patient's blood pressure is 175/89 mmHg, up from 152/87 mmHg; heart rate is 70 bpm, down from 90 bpm; oxygen saturation is 95% at baseline; and temperature is 99.5°F (37.5°C). The nurse's first priority is to:

    A. Assess the patient's blood glucose.
    B. Notify the doctor and request an order to obtain an EKG.
    C. Put icepacks in the patient's armpits and reassess temperature in 15 minutes.
    D. Assist the patient with sitting upright and to the side of the bed.

16. A patient is admitted from the ED with a diagnosis of hemorrhagic stroke. Which of the following interventions should the nurse implement to prevent rebleeding?

    A. Encourage bed rest and supine positioning.
    B. Administer stool softeners.
    C. Administer aspirin to prevent clots.
    D. Do not turn the patient.

(See answers next page.)

13. D) "Those changes would help to reduce the risk factors for developing another stroke; however, speak with your physician before you stop taking your medications."

Therapeutic communication is essential when conducting patient teaching; therefore, educating the patient on risk factors and answering the question are most appropriate. Regardless of whether the nurse has educated them on risk factors, telling patients they can stop their medications is not within the nursing scope of practice. Offering to contact the physician disregards the patient's question; the nurse should be able to respond appropriately to the question within the scope of nursing practice.

14. B) "It's normal to feel this way after a stroke. The goal of physical therapy is to help you get as close to your normal self as possible."

The use of therapeutic communication is essential when speaking to patients; therefore, acknowledging the patient's feelings and educating on the purpose of rehabilitation is the most therapeutic response. Telling the patient not to worry disregards the patient's feelings. Suggesting contact with a psychologist is not a therapeutic communication technique. Telling the patient "Everything will be fine" is false reassurance and disregards the patient's feelings.

15. D) Assist the patient with sitting upright and to the side of the bed.

Autonomic dysreflexia (AD) is a potential medical emergency that occurs in patients with spinal cord injuries at T6 or above. It is characterized by a sudden increase in blood pressure (more than 20 mmHg) and severe migraines, and it can result in facial flushing and heart rate irregularity. The immediate priority for the nurse is to sit the patient at a 90-degree angle and, if possible, allow the legs to dangle to help reduce the blood pressure. Assessing the patient's blood glucose and obtaining an EKG are not appropriate interventions. Placing icepacks in the armpits and reassessing the problem in 15 minutes will result in more patient harm.

16. B) Administer stool softeners.

The priority nursing intervention after a hemorrhagic stroke is to prevent rebleeding. Patients should be instructed to avoid Valsalva maneuvers, so administering stool softeners is an appropriate intervention. Patients should be instructed to keep the head of bed elevated between 15 and 30 degrees, as supine positioning is contraindicated. Aspirin should never be given to patients who have had a hemorrhagic stroke, because it can cause more bleeding and lead to further damage. There is no contraindication to turning patients with hemorrhagic stroke.

17. During discharge teaching for a patient with a spinal cord injury, the nurse discusses autonomic dysreflexia (AD) as a potential complication. The patient's wife asks, "What should I do if I think he's experiencing AD?" Which response is most appropriate?

   A. "You should have him lie down to decrease his anxiety."
   B. "You should perform a straight catheterization."
   C. "You should administer his antihypertensives."
   D. "You should assess his blood sugar."

18. A patient is transferred to a surgical unit with a spinal cord injury at C4. The nurse includes all of the following interventions in the care plan EXCEPT:

   A. Implement bowel management protocol.
   B. Perform intermittent catheterization frequently.
   C. Administer acetaminophen as needed for headaches.
   D. Immediately lay the patient flat to reduce blood pressure.

19. The nurse is reviewing the care plan for a patient diagnosed with myasthenia gravis. The nurse includes all of the following interventions in the care plan EXCEPT:

   A. Administer cholinesterase inhibitors (physostigmine) and ensure proper dosing/ timing.
   B. Monitor feeding time intervals and ensure proper nutrition.
   C. Schedule medication times 30 to 45 minutes prior to meal preparation or feeding times.
   D. Drink caffeine and alcohol in moderation.

20. The nurse is caring for a patient admitted for cholinergic crisis, with a history of myasthenia gravis. Which assessment findings would indicate that the patient is now in a myasthenic crisis?

   A. Tachycardia
   B. Bradycardia
   C. Vomiting
   D. Hypotension

21. The nurse is reviewing discharge medication with a male patient diagnosed with Parkinson's disease and his wife. Which statement made by the wife would indicate that the nurse's teaching regarding the drug carbidopa–levodopa is effective?

   A. "I will make sure he takes the medicine with meals and at the scheduled time."
   B. "I'm optimistic that the medicine will decrease absorption of dopamine and improve his balance."
   C. "I will look for an improvement in his urinary symptoms."
   D. "Now that this medicine will enhance his visual acuity, he can resume driving."

(See answers next page.)

17. B) "You should perform a straight catheterization."

AD can cause an imbalance in the autonomic system, resulting in life-threatening hypertension if the precipitating cause goes unnoticed. The priority will be to sit the patient upright and assess for the precipitating cause, such as a full bladder or bowel. Performing a straight catheterization to empty the bladder is likely the most appropriate response. Although lying down will decrease anxiety, causative factors should be addressed. Antihypertensives and assessing the blood sugar are interventions that may be warranted after the precipitating cause is removed.

18. D) Immediately lay the patient flat to reduce blood pressure.

The patient's spinal cord was injured at C4, which is above T6, placing the patient at increased risk for developing autonomic dysreflexia (AD). The first sign of AD is severe hypertension. Priority interventions should be aimed at reducing the patient's blood pressure and assessing for precipitating causes, such as a full bowel or bladder. Patients should sit upright to reduce blood pressure orthostatically, so it is not appropriate to lay the patient flat. Severe headaches are another sign of AD, so administering acetaminophen as needed for headaches is warranted. Assessing for the precipitating cause, such as a full bladder or bowel, is an appropriate intervention.

19. D) Drink caffeine and alcohol in moderation.

Myasthenia gravis is a chronic, progressive autoimmune disorder that results in decreased acetylcholine activity in the synapses. This disorder is exacerbated by triggers, such as alcohol and caffeine, so patients should completely refrain from drinking either substance. All other interventions are appropriate for the management of a patient with myasthenia gravis.

20. A) Tachycardia

A myasthenic crisis typically results from under-medication in the synapses, which results in tachycardia and hypertension. Bradycardia, hypotension, and vomiting are likely findings associated with a cholinergic crisis.

21. C) "I will look for an improvement in his urinary symptoms."

Patients who are diagnosed with Parkinson's disease can experience dysfunctions within their autonomic nervous system, which can lead to urinary incontinence, urgency, and frequency; therefore, teaching is effective when the wife is aware that an improvement in urinary symptoms should occur. Levodopa should be taken 30 minutes to 1 hour prior to meals on an empty stomach; taking with meals indicates ineffective teaching. The medicine will increase, not decrease, the absorption of dopamine. The medicine will not enhance visual acuity.

22. A patient is admitted for recurring migraines. The physician orders a cerebral angiogram. Which statement best describes the purpose of this procedure?

    A. A cerebral angiogram detects nystagmus, which may identify problems with the cerebellar system.

    B. A cerebral angiogram identifies the size, shape, and location of intracranial structures and any shifts.

    C. A cerebral angiogram is done to detect narrowing or blockages within a blood vessel.

    D. A cerebral angiogram detects spinal cord lesions and nerve root compression.

23. The nurse is caring for a male patient diagnosed with advanced Parkinson's disease (PD). Which assessment finding should the nurse anticipate?

    A. Memory loss

    B. Bradykinesia

    C. Gaze paralysis

    D. Muscle flaccidity

24. A patient with a solitary tumor in the brain has dysphagia. The nurse contacts the speech therapist to evaluate the patient based on knowledge that which cranial nerve is affected?

    A. IX

    B. VII

    C. V

    D. VI

25. The caregiver of an 80-year-old male patient diagnosed with Alzheimer's disease asks, "How do patients get this disease?" Which response is MOST appropriate for the nurse to provide?

    A. "Some risk factors associated with Alzheimer's disease are advanced age and family history."

    B. "This disease can develop after long-term exposure to environmental toxins such as herbicides and pesticides."

    C. "If you live in close proximity to industrial or chemical plants, you may be at increased risk."

    D. "Patients who are heavy smokers and drug users are at increased risk for developing Alzheimer's disease due to the damaging effects to the nervous system."

26. Which statement best describes amyotrophic lateral sclerosis (ALS)?

    A. ALS is a progressive degenerative disorder that involves the destruction of spinal cord and cranial motor nerves.

    B. ALS is a progressive degenerative disease that affects the myelin sheath found in the central nervous system neurons.

    C. ALS is a chronic, progressive, hereditary disease that results in memory loss and uncontrolled movements.

    D. ALS is an autoimmune disorder characterized by skeletal muscle weakness and fatigue that worsens with exercise.

(See answers next page.)

22. C) A cerebral angiogram is done to detect narrowing or blockages within a blood vessel.

A cerebral angiogram is done to detect bulging, narrowing, or blockages within the blood vessels. During the procedure, a dye is injected into a vein for visualization of blood vessels on a monitor. An electronystagmography (ENG) detects nystagmus. A CT scan is done to visualize intracranial structures for size, shape, location, and shifts. A myelography is done to detect spinal cord lesions and nerve root compression.

23. B) Bradykinesia

Bradykinesia, or slow movement, is considered one of the cardinal signs of PD. Patients who are diagnosed with advanced PD do not have memory loss, but they may have difficulty with vocal articulation. Visual disturbances, such as gaze paralysis, are common in patients with multiple sclerosis, not in PD. Muscle rigidity, not flaccidity, is a cardinal sign of PD.

24. A) IX

Cranial nerve IX (glossopharyngeal) is the major nerve for the swallowing center, along with cranial nerves X (vagus) and XII (hypoglossal). If the patient is having dysphagia, the tumor could be affecting one of these cranial nerves. Cranial nerve VII (facial) affects the sensory abilities of the tongue, such as taste. Cranial nerve V (trigeminal) controls the sensory and motor ability of the face and eyes. Cranial nerve VI (abducens) controls the motor function of the eye.

25. A) "Some risk factors associated with Alzheimer's disease are advanced age and family history."

Alzheimer's disease is a chronic, progressive, neurologic degenerative disorder that results in cognitive, intellectual, and behavioral impairments. Risk factors are advancing age and family history. Environmental toxins and living in close proximity to chemical plants describe the risk factors associated Parkinson's disease. Being a heavy smoker and drug user increases a patient's risk for developing a cerebrovascular accident.

26. A) ALS is a progressive degenerative disorder that involves the destruction of spinal cord and cranial motor nerves.

ALS is a disease that involves the destruction of anterior horn cells and corticospinal tracts in the brainstem that affect the cranial motor nerves and spinal cord. Multiple sclerosis affects the myelin sheath in neurons found in the central nervous system. Huntington disease is characterized by memory loss and involuntary movement. Myasthenia gravis is a disease that affects the skeletal muscle system, resulting in weakness and fatigue that worsens with exercise and improves with rest.

27. The nurse is caring for a patient admitted with an exacerbation of multiple sclerosis. Which of these assessment findings would indicate a medical emergency?

    A. Difficulty picking up things
    B. Frequent swallowing and coughing
    C. Fatigue
    D. Ptosis

(See answers next page.)

27. B) Frequent swallowing and coughing

Patients who are diagnosed with multiple sclerosis are at risk for aspiration pneumonia, due to damage to the nerves that control chewing and swallowing. Frequent swallowing and coughing could be signs of aspiration. Difficulty picking up things is a common occurrence in patients with multiple sclerosis. Although fatigue and visual disturbances may occur, these are expected clinical findings and do not indicate a medical emergency.

Eyes, Ears, Nose, and Throat

1. The nurse is assigned to a total laryngectomy patient who is on postoperative day 2. During morning medication administration, the nurse finds the patient unresponsive. The nurse calls the emergency response team and initiates chest compressions. Which of the following actions should the nurse perform next to aid in resuscitation?

   A. Provide rescue ventilations via mouth-to-mouth with a barrier device at a 30:2 ratio.
   B. Provide rescue ventilation via bag valve mask to mouth every 8 to 10 seconds.
   C. Provide rescue breath via bag valve mask to stoma at a 15:2 ratio.
   D. Provide rescue ventilation via bag valve mask to stoma every 6 seconds.

2. Which of the following precautions is MOST appropriate for the nurse to include in the care plan of a patient with Ménière's disease?

   A. Fall precautions
   B. Seizure precautions
   C. Neutropenic precautions
   D. Bleeding precautions

3. What is the priority nursing intervention to promote healing immediately after eye surgery?

   A. Encourage the patient to drink plenty of fluids.
   B. Encourage the patient to lie in a semi-Fowler's position.
   C. Offer the patient a warm compress to apply over the surgical site.
   D. Encourage the patient to lie in a supine position and reduce the lighting.

4. Which of the following statements, if made by the patient, indicates a correct understanding of how to instill eye drops?

   A. "I rub my eyes after each eye drop."
   B. "My doctor prescribed me two different eye drops. I typically instill them at the same time so that I don't forget."
   C. "I always have to squeeze the bottle to get the medicine to fall out."
   D. "I try to avoid contaminating the eye dispenser at all times."

1. D) Provide rescue ventilation via bag valve mask to stoma every 6 seconds.

A total laryngectomy involves a complete separation of the upper airway from the lower airway, resulting in a neck stoma. The stoma site at the neck becomes the new airway; therefore rescue breath ventilation via mouth-to-mouth is ineffective. Ventilation breaths should be provided every 6 seconds at the stoma site; thus, every 8 to 10 seconds is incorrect. Ventilation breaths via bag valve mask at a 15:2 ratio is the resuscitation rate for a child.

2. A) Fall precautions

Patients diagnosed with Ménière's disease can have sudden episodes of vertigo, tinnitus, and a sensorineural hearing loss, placing them at increased risk for falls. Seizure precautions are unrelated to the problem. Neutropenic precautions are unwarranted unless the patient is immunocompromised. Patients with Ménière's disease do not require bleeding precautions, so this is not the most appropriate response.

3. B) Encourage the patient to lie in a semi-Fowler's position.

The priority goal after eye surgery is patient safety and prevention of complications. Elevating the head of the bed and reducing the lighting can reduce intraocular pressure. Although it is important to drink fluids, this is not the priority action to promote healing. Applying a warm compress over the surgical site is a long-term recovery recommendation; it is not done in the immediate acute phase. Postoperative eye surgery patients should not lie supine because this can increase intraocular pressure.

4. D) "I try to avoid contaminating the eye dispenser at all times."

The instillation of eye drops must be done carefully to avoid contamination, which can lead to eye infections. It is not recommended for patients to rub their eyes after instilling eye drops to avoid displacing the medication. When administering multiple eye drops, patients should always wait 5 to 15 minutes before instilling the second medication. To avoid over-medicating, patients should not squeeze the bottle when instilling the medication.

5. A patient has returned to the room after having cataract eye surgery. Twelve hours later, the patient suddenly begins to complain of black spots floating in the left visual field. The most appropriate next action for the nurse is to:

   A. Notify the physician immediately, because the patient could have a retinal detachment.
   B. Do nothing, because this is an expected finding after this procedure.
   C. Contact the physician to obtain an order for dorzolamide.
   D. Continue to monitor because this could indicate a complication.

6. The nurse is teaching a patient about discharge medications. The patient is prescribed atropine ophthalmic solution (atropine sulfate) for both eyes. During the teaching, the patient asks, "Is it okay for me to drive to work after instilling this medication?" Which of the following responses would be most appropriate to give to the patient?

   A. "You can drive but only for short distances because this medication can cause diplopia."
   B. "You should not drive a car immediately after instilling this medication because it can cause blurry vision."
   C. "You should not drive a car for at least 15 minutes after instilling this medication because it can cause dizziness."
   D. "You should omit the eye drops if you plan to drive that day."

7. Which of the following interventions should be included in the care plan for a patient who underwent nasal cautery for epistaxis?

   A. Encourage the patient to limit fluid intake.
   B. Encourage the patient to lie flat in the event of nosebleeds after surgery.
   C. Encourage the patient to blow the nose frequently to reduce congestion.
   D. Encourage the patient to use a prescribed nasal spray several times a day.

(See answers next page.)

5. A) Notify the physician immediately, because the patient could have a retinal detachment.

Bleeding occurs as a result of retinal detachment, which manifests as black spots or floaters in the eye. Retinal detachment is not an expected finding but rather a complication of cataract eye surgery. Dorzolamide is an eye medication used to treat glaucoma and reduce pressure in the eye; therefore, it is not the next best action. It is not appropriate for the nurse to continue monitoring for a complication because the patient is experiencing retinal detachment, which should be reported to the physician immediately.

6. B) "You should not drive a car immediately after instilling this medication because it can cause blurry vision."

Atropine sulfate is an anticholinergic medication that causes the pupils to dilate and the eye muscles to relax, resulting in blurry vision and sensitivity to light. Patients should not operate machinery or drive while taking this medication. Diplopia and dizziness are not side effects of atropine sulfate. The patient should plan activities around the use of the medication, but the eye drops should not be omitted.

7. D) Encourage the patient to use a prescribed nasal spray several times a day.

Nasal cautery is a surgical procedure performed to prevent epistaxis (nosebleeds). After the procedure, patients are prescribed an antibacterial saline nasal spray or ointment to keep the nasal mucosa moist. To help with recovery, fluid intake should not be limited after surgery, but instead encouraged. Patients should refrain from lying flat in order to prevent blood from entering the posterior pharynx and increasing the risk for aspiration. Patients should not blow the nose for 2 weeks after surgery, because doing so can dislodge the formed clot.

Integumentary System

1. A patient who sustained full-thickness burns over the entire lower body is admitted to the medical–surgical unit from the ED. The main goal of treatment 48 hours after this type of burn injury is to:

   A. Encourage ambulation.
   B. Replace fluid loss.
   C. Provide psychosocial care.
   D. Administer pain medications.

2. Which of the following patients is more likely to develop a pressure injury?

   A. An 87-year-old male with obesity who is confused and incontinent
   B. A 24-year-old male who is postoperative day 1 from a laparoscopic cholecystectomy
   C. A 45-year-old female with obesity who is postoperative day 0 from a unilateral oophorectomy
   D. A 66-year-old female who is immobile and not able to tolerate food by mouth

3. Which of these comments, if made by a patient, would indicate a knowledge deficit regarding the prevention of squamous cell carcinoma?

   A. "I will be sure to monitor my skin frequently for lesions and changes in color."
   B. "I'm concerned about a mole on my shoulder."
   C. "I no longer use tanning salons because the natural sunlight is better for my vitamin D absorption."
   D. "I typically wear protective clothing and sunscreen when I'm at the park with my family."

4. Which of the following interventions is NOT recommended for the prevention of pressure ulcers?

   A. Use of diapers
   B. Frequent turning
   C. Proper nutrition
   D. Reducing friction

1. B) Replace fluid loss.

In the acute phase 48 to 72 hours after a major burn injury, the top priority is life support. Fluid resuscitation is key to prevent hypovolemic shock in patients with major burn injuries. Although it is important to encourage ambulation and offer psychosocial support, this is likely not the priority in the acute phase of a burn injury. Full-thickness burns that extend through the dermis and epidermis are typically painless; however, this can vary with each person.

2. D) A 66-year-old female who is immobile and not able to tolerate food by mouth

Patients are at increased risk for developing a pressure injury when they are immobile and have poor nutrition. An 87-year-old male with obesity who is confused and incontinent might develop incontinence-associated dermatitis, but incontinence is not a leading cause of pressure injury development. Postoperative patients are at increased risk for developing pressure injuries if they are immobile for an extended period of time, but this is likely not the case in patients who undergo laparoscopic and/or minor procedures.

3. C) "I no longer use tanning salons because the natural sunlight is better for my vitamin D absorption."

Squamous cell carcinoma is caused by prolonged sun exposure and the use of tanning beds or exposure to UV light. It is recommended for patients to frequently assess their skin and monitor for changes. It is important for patients to understand interventions aimed at reducing the risk factors for skin cancer, such as the use of sunscreen and protective clothing.

4. A) Use of diapers

The use of diapers or multiple underpads can lead to the development of pressure injuries. Frequent turning, proper nutrition, and reducing friction are all recommended as interventions to prevent pressure injuries.

5. A patient is transferred to a medical unit from a long-term care facility. Upon patient assessment, the nurse notices that the patient has a large wound to the sacrum. The wound measures about 4 cm by 5 cm, with an unknown depth. The wound bed is covered with slough. What type of pressure injury would the nurse characterize this as?

   A. Unstageable pressure injury
   B. Stage 4
   C. Deep tissue pressure injury
   D. Stage 3

6. In the absence of a wound care nurse's recommendation, what would be the most appropriate conservative treatment for a patient admitted to the medical–surgical unit with a stage 4 pressure injury?

   A. Hydrocolloid dressing
   B. Dry dressing
   C. Wet-to-dry dressing
   D. Hydrogel dressing

(See answers next page.)

5. A) Unstageable pressure injury

Pressure injuries are characterized by the depth of injury to the skin. With unstageable pressure injuries, the extent of tissue injury is not ascertainable because the wound bed is covered with slough or eschar. In a stage 3 or 4 pressure injury, the extent of tissue damage is exposed. With a deep tissue injury, the skin may be intact or nonintact with a localized area of nonblanchable dark red, maroon, or purple discoloration that may also manifest as a blood-filled blister.

6. C) Wet-to-dry dressing

A wet-to-dry dressing is the most appropriate conservative treatment for a stage 4 pressure injury. Hydrocolloid dressings are recommended for clean stage 2 and shallow stage 3 pressure injuries. Dry dressings are not recommended because they can cause more tissue damage. Hydrogel dressings are recommended for shallow, minimally exudating wounds.

Part II
Practice Exams

MSNCB Certification Practice Exam

1. The nurse is caring for an adult patient with an acute kidney injury (AKI). The patient weighs 145 lb (66 kg) and has a urine output of less than 400 mL/24 hr. What phase of AKI does this suggest?

   A. Recovery
   B. Diuretic
   C. Onset
   D. Oliguric

2. The nurse is assessing a patient for musculoskeletal abnormalities with a physical therapist. The patient walks with a staggering, uncoordinated gait that has a sway. The nurse identifies this gait as:

   A. Festinating.
   B. Spastic.
   C. Ataxic.
   D. Steppage.

3. Which finding will the nurse expect when monitoring a patient with polycystic kidney disease (PKD)?

   A. No pain
   B. Hypotension
   C. Hematuria
   D. Nonpalpable kidneys

4. Which action will the nurse take when noticing that a patient with Alzheimer's disease has become agitated and confused?

   A. Encourage the patient to go for a ride with a family member.
   B. Provide family photos and familiar objects to the patient.
   C. Allow the patient to follow their own schedule for toileting.
   D. Speak as if the patient were in their childhood years.

5. What action should the nurse should take when receiving a telephone order from a provider?

   A. Immediately carry out the order.
   B. Write down the order and then read it back to the provider.
   C. Write the order in the patient's medical record immediately.
   D. Remind the provider that telephone orders are not permitted.

6. The nurse is providing education about the use of isotretinoin to a patient who has severe acne. Which adverse effect will the nurse educate the patient to report immediately?

    A. Pruritus
    B. Depressed thoughts
    C. Increased frequency of sunburn
    D. Stomach upset

7. The nurse has been asked to help establish an evidence-based policy on alarm use for the unit's telemetric monitors. When gathering information on which to base the policy, the nurse should refer to:

    A. Peer-reviewed journals.
    B. Online discussion groups.
    C. Nursing textbooks.
    D. Research articles in prepublication form.

8. A patient who was scheduled for amputation of the right great toe secondary to a diabetic ulcer comes to the recovery room with an amputation of the left great toe. The patient's spouse is at the bedside and asks the nurse for the reason for the left-sided amputation. No additional information has been provided to the nurse at this time. Which principle should the nurse employ when discussing the patient's procedure with the spouse?

    A. Do not assume responsibility for disclosure before speaking to the provider.
    B. Deny any possibility of a sentinel event to the patient and the spouse.
    C. Do not discuss any concerns about the incident with the provider.
    D. Refer the patient and the spouse to the facility's ombuds.

9. The measure that most effectively reduces the overall risk of healthcare-associated infections is:

    A. Always wearing a mask when caring for patients.
    B. Providing annual influenza vaccinations.
    C. Performing consistent hand hygiene.
    D. Keeping employee health records up to date.

10. The nurse is planning a teaching session for a female patient who has been diagnosed with a urinary tract infection (UTI). The nurse should teach:

    A. Force yourself to urinate every hour.
    B. Urinate after sexual intercourse.
    C. Stop taking the antibiotic when symptoms improve.
    D. Limit fluid intake to avoid the urge to urinate.

11. A patient with type 1 diabetes has been admitted with a diagnosis of diabetic ketoacidosis (DKA). What finding would the nurse expect to be present?

    A. Hypernatremia
    B. Normal serum potassium
    C. Slightly rapid respirations
    D. Hyperventilation

12. A patient with calcium oxalate renal calculi is preparing to be discharged. The nurse will provide nutrition education that includes:

    A. Limiting fiber intake.
    B. Reducing the intake of protein.
    C. Increasing sodium intake.
    D. Adopting a low-calcium diet.

13. A patient presents with diaphoresis, jitters, and palpitations approximately 90 minutes after taking their morning insulin. The initial intervention that is most appropriate for this patient is:

    A. Schedule a blood glucose check in 1 hour.
    B. Change the insulin administration time.
    C. Educate the patient on a proper diabetic diet.
    D. Administer a simple carbohydrate to the patient.

14. A patient reports weight gain, impaired memory, and fatigue. On assessment, vital signs are blood pressure of 120/72 mmHg, pulse rate of 56 beats/min, respiratory rate of 18 breaths/min, and temperature of 98.4°F (36.9°C). The provider suspects primary hypothyroidism. The nurse knows the lab result that is most consistent with a diagnosis of hypothyroidism is:

    A. Low thyroid-stimulating hormone (TSH).
    B. Normal total T4.
    C. Low free T3.
    D. High free T4.

15. A patient complaining of muscle weakness, anorexia with weight loss, and darkening of the skin is suspected of having Addison's disease. Which lab result does the nurse recognize as the most diagnostic of the suspected condition?

    A. Normal potassium level
    B. Hyperglycemia
    C. High cortisol level
    D. Hyponatremia

16. A patient has thick, reddened patches of skin covered by silver-white scales on both elbows. The nurse explains to the patient that these findings are most closely associated with:

    A. Scabies.
    B. Seborrhea.
    C. Psoriasis.
    D. Squamous cell carcinoma.

17. The nurse is caring for a patient who is suspected of having polycystic kidney disease. The nurse knows that the diagnostic study that would be most beneficial in diagnosing the condition is:

    A. Hemoglobin A1C.
    B. Abdominal CT scan.
    C. Complete blood count (CBC) and basic metabolic panel (BMP).
    D. Renal sonography.

18. What finding would alert the nurse that a patient may be at increased risk for urinary incontinence?

    A. Dizziness
    B. Restricted mobility
    C. Pruritis
    D. Petechiae

19. During a health history, the statement by a patient that would indicate a risk of renal calculi is:

    A. "I'm really bad about staying hydrated."
    B. "I've had more stress since we adopted our child last year."
    C. "I've been exercising more than usual."
    D. "I've been drinking a lot of orange juice lately."

20. Nursing management for treatment of acute poststreptococcal glomerulonephritis would include:

    A. Recommending increased activity.
    B. Increasing sodium and fluid intake.
    C. Providing education on peritoneal dialysis.
    D. Limiting dietary protein intake.

21. A patient with acute kidney injury (AKI) is being assessed to determine whether the cause of the AKI is prerenal, renal, or postrenal. If the cause is prerenal, the condition that most likely caused it is:

    A. Aminoglycoside toxicity.
    B. Ureterolithiasis.
    C. Renal carcinoma.
    D. Sepsis.

22. The nurse understands that an overall goal for the patient being treated for osteoarthritis (OA) is to:

    A. Reverse joint damage and regain function.
    B. Promote self-care independence.
    C. Eliminate pain with physical activities.
    D. Correct the appearance of bony abnormalities.

23. Which test is the most accurate way to diagnose pulmonary hypertension?

    A. EKG
    B. Chest x-ray
    C. CT scan
    D. Cardiac catheterization

24. What term refers to the condition in which the skin loses its pigment cells (melanocytes), resulting in discolored patches on different areas of the body?

    A. Alopecia
    B. Telangiectasia
    C. Vitiligo
    D. Lichenification

25. The nurse is teaching a patient about the correct storage and proper use of nitroglycerin. Which statement by the patient demonstrates the need for further education?

    A. "I understand that I should keep the medication close to me at all times."
    B. "I know that the medication should be kept refrigerated at all times."
    C. "I can repeat the dose every 5 minutes if I need to."
    D. "I should replace the medication every 6 months."

26. A patient presents to the ED after being stung by a bee. The patient reports difficulty swallowing, tightness in the throat, congestion, and hoarseness of the voice. The medication that will be immediately administered is:

    A. Epinephrine 1:1,000, 0.3 mL to 0.5 mL intramuscularly (IM) or intravenously (IV).
    B. Prednisone, 4 mg by mouth.
    C. Diphenhydramine, 25 to 50 mg IM or IV.
    D. Famotidine, 20 mg by mouth.

27. Which intervention would the ICU nurse anticipate when caring for a patient with acute thyrotoxicosis?

    A. Administer medications that increase thyroid hormone production.
    B. Provide monitoring for dysrhythmias and decompensation.
    C. Auscultate lung sounds and reduce the rate of oxygenation.
    D. Limit administration of intravenous dexamethasone to a single dose.

28. What instructions would be provided upon discharge to a patient admitted for diabetic ketoacidosis?

    A. "Check your blood sugar at least every 3 to 4 hours."
    B. "Restrict the amount of oral fluids to prevent overload."
    C. "Eat several high-fiber small meals throughout the day, according to hunger."
    D. "Expect your temperature to be slightly lower than normal for 1 to 2 weeks after discharge."

29. Atrial fibrillation can cause which neurologic condition?

   A. Traumatic brain injury
   B. Parkinson's disease
   C. Hemorrhagic stroke
   D. Embolic stroke

30. The nurse suspects that a patient with a fractured radius has compartment syndrome. What physical exam finding would be consistent with the suspected diagnosis?

   A. Pain in the arm increases when the arm is allowed to hang in a dependent position.
   B. Pain in the arm resolves with full flexion or extension of the arm.
   C. Pain in the arm worsens when the arm is positioned at the level of the shoulder.
   D. Pain radiates up the arm to the scapula when the patient lies supine.

31. The most common cause of basal cell carcinoma is:

   A. Burns.
   B. Immunosuppression.
   C. Chronic sun exposure.
   D. Radiation exposure.

32. What initial teaching should the nurse include for a patient newly diagnosed with moderate hypertension?

   A. Instruct the patient to contact the provider every time their blood pressure is elevated on readings at home.
   B. Educate the patient on the dietary approaches to stop hypertension (DASH) diet and the importance of regular exercise.
   C. Encourage the patient to reduce salt consumption and to limit fluid intake to no more than 1,500 mL/d.
   D. Advise the patient that an urgent cardiology referral is needed at this time to evaluate their hypertension.

33. Which disorder results from a lack of clotting factors?

   A. Thrombocytopenia
   B. Thalassemia
   C. Sickle cell anemia
   D. Hemophilia

34. The nurse has been notified that an otherwise healthy adult with no history of hypertension has a current blood pressure of 192/80 mmHg. What intervention should the nurse complete first?

   A. Recheck the blood pressure manually in both arms.
   B. Assess the patient for signs and symptoms of heart disease.
   C. Document in the chart and recheck the blood pressure in 4 hours.
   D. Administer pain medication to lower the blood pressure.

35. The nurse is caring for a patient with a history of diabetes. The provider has ordered oral corticosteroid therapy for the treatment of bronchitis. What will be the first action taken by the nurse?

    A. Contact the medical provider and clarify the orders.
    B. Maintain the home glycemic regimen without change.
    C. Provide a simple carbohydrate snack with administration.
    D. Implement blood-sugar checks every 2 hours.

36. When educating a patient on the use of immediate-release metformin, how will the nurse describe the expected action of the medication?

    A. There is a 4-week time frame for optimal effects.
    B. The duration of action depends on liver metabolism.
    C. The half-life of the medication is 48 hours.
    D. Peak effects are seen within 2 to 3 hours.

37. The process of hyperaldosteronism development will affect what body function?

    A. Excretion of urinary waste
    B. Blood perfusion to the alveoli of the lungs
    C. Digestion of food and absorption of nutrients
    D. Fluid and electrolyte balance

38. When administering the influenza vaccination to a patient, the nurse will:

    A. Educate the patient on the vaccine, including desired outcomes and possible side effects.
    B. Premedicate the patient with acetaminophen or ibuprofen to prevent fever.
    C. Explain the injection site may be discolored, painful, and swollen for 4 to 5 days.
    D. Explain that the vaccine should be repeated if they have an acute influenza episode.

39. When caring for a patient after surgery who has a history of long-term corticosteroid use, the best course of action to address the patient's compromised immunity and prevent the associated complications is to:

    A. Educate on measures of infection prevention and handwashing.
    B. Educate on mechanism of action of corticosteroid therapy and its potential side effects.
    C. Review the antibiotic regimen and discuss how it will prevent infection.
    D. Encourage earlier ambulation and mobility toward recovery.

40. What action would be taken first to address a patient's report of back pain associated with urination?

    A. Obtain a urine sample on the next void.
    B. Encourage the patient to drink more fluids.
    C. Perform a musculoskeletal examination.
    D. Educate the patient on hygiene practices.

41. A patient with kidney failure who is undergoing hemodialysis is asking about the cause of anemia. What statement by the nurse will address the patient's concern?

    A. "The kidneys are responsible for maintaining the number of circulating red blood cells."

    B. "Your low-phosphorus diet is the cause of the anemia, but we will continue to monitor you."

    C. "Your kidneys are not producing enough erythropoietin, which helps your body make red blood cells."

    D. "Anemia is a result of bone marrow dysfunction and is not related to your condition."

42. An older male patient reports painful urination with abdominal pain and inability to void at times. What is the next step the nurse should take in the care of this patient?

    A. Encourage the patient to increase fluid intake.

    B. Recommend the use of condoms with intercourse

    C. Perform a full abdominal examination.

    D. Ask the patient whether he has perianal or rectal pain.

43. Upon entering the room of a patient who has received peritoneal dialysis, the nurse observes an acute change in the patient's mental status. What will be the first action by the nurse?

    A. Obtain consent for an emergency hemodialysis treatment.

    B. Assess vital signs and maintain the safety of the room environment.

    C. Document the assessment findings and implement frequent safety checks.

    D. Administer preordered insulin based on the glucose content of the peritoneal dialysis fluid used.

44. What is the most appropriate element of care to be discussed when educating a hospitalized patient diagnosed with muscular dystrophy on fall prevention?

    A. "Using all four side rails is considered a restraint, so we will line the bed with pillows to provide a barrier and prevent falls."

    B. "To prevent falling at night, I recommend that you urinate in the absorbent pads in the bed rather than go to the restroom."

    C. "Your call bell should be located next to you at all times, so you can ask for help when you are getting out of bed."

    D. "To prevent infection, you must maintain the same level of independence while hospitalized that you had at home."

45. What is the most important daily care plan intervention used by the nurse to help prevent complications in a patient with quadriplegia?

    A. Schedule repositioning of the patient every 2 hours.

    B. Recommend a minimum of 2 hours of sunlight a day.

    C. Encourage the patient to have meals in the dining room.

    D. Check the temperature of the legs each time vital signs are obtained.

46. What is the immediate nursing action when caring for a patient with a history of migraine headaches who reports new onset of visual disturbances?

    A. Maintain an environment free from bright lights.
    B. Provide acetaminophen for the patient's headache.
    C. Educate the patient on the importance of balancing rest with activities and drinking plenty of fluids.
    D. Report findings to the medical provider and await new orders.

47. A patient is admitted after sustaining extensive skin burns to the torso and lower extremities 4 hours ago. During this initial period, the nurse will prepare for the most common complication by:

    A. Measuring accurate intake and output values.
    B. Changing burn dressings frequently.
    C. Preparing the patient for a possible skin graft in the future.
    D. Educating the caregiver on technique of dressing changes.

48. What is the initial nursing action when receiving an order for a phenytoin level lab test for a patient diagnosed with epilepsy?

    A. Schedule the test for bedtime after all scheduled doses have been administered.
    B. Check the current dose and administration schedule for the medication.
    C. Educate the patient on the need to fast for 8 hours before the lab test.
    D. Immediately obtain the blood specimen and submit to the lab.

49. What information will the nurse include when teaching the patient about skin discolorations caused by radiation therapy?

    A. Changes to the skin will not resolve completely when therapy is stopped; some discoloration may remain.
    B. The discolored sites will be painful during treatment but will return to normal upon completion of therapy.
    C. Skin moisturizer should be applied daily to prevent the skin discolorations from becoming permanent.
    D. Itching in the affected area will resolve after treatment stops, but changes to the skin color may not.

50. A patient whose gastric output is noted to be red in color is also reporting lightheadedness. What is the immediate action by the nurse?

    A. Clamp the gastric tube, and then reassess the gastric output and vital signs in 1 hour.
    B. Reposition the patient in bed, assess the vital signs, and measure amount of gastric output.
    C. Notify the patient's emergency contact, and obtain values for intake and output.
    D. Elevate the head of the bed slightly and assist with coughing and deep breathing.

51. A patient admitted to the unit suddenly reports sharp, excruciating pain in the right lower quadrant that is worse with any change in position. The immediate action by the nurse will be to:

    A. Administer a laxative as needed and reassess in 1 hour.
    B. Review medical records for pain medication orders.
    C. Perform abdominal assessment and report findings to the provider.
    D. Educate the patient on nonpharmacologic pain-relief techniques.

52. While eating lunch, a patient develops sudden difficulty swallowing and is noted to have weakness on the left side. The nurse's priority action is to:

    A. Activate the rapid response team and call the medical provider about the status change.
    B. Reposition the patient and assess the gag reflex and reaction to light.
    C. Review the medical record to check for any medications that may be causing the symptoms.
    D. Measure intake and output values and reposition the patient to semi-Fowler's position.

53. A patient visits a clinic and reports difficulty swallowing. On physical assessment, the nurse observes sores in the mouth. The patient states that a saliva substitute is taken for dry mouth. The healthcare provider recommends a biopsy to assess for oral cancer. While awaiting results from the biopsy, the nurse would instruct the patient to:

    A. Add spicy seasonings to food.
    B. Use a thickening agent for liquids.
    C. Discontinue use of the saliva substitute.
    D. Avoid frequent rinsing of the mouth.

54. A patient is admitted with hematemesis, pyrosis, stomach pain, and singultus. A healthcare provider conducts a biopsy, diagnoses the patient with stomach cancer, and recommends radiation therapy for treatment. After several days of treatment, the patient is being discharged. The nurse's discharge teaching will include instructions to:

    A. Drink water with meals.
    B. Avoid lying flat after eating.
    C. Avoid commercial mouthwashes.
    D. Eat soft, bland, nonacidic foods.

55. A patient reports rectal bleeding and mild fever. The patient's clinical history involves deep vein thrombosis, for which the patient takes warfarin, and chronic headaches managed with aspirin. The provider recommends a guaiac fecal occult blood test. The nurse explains the necessary precautions to be taken before the test. The nurse knows that patient teaching has been effective when the patient states:

    A. "I can eat raw melon, turnips, and radishes before the scheduled test."
    B. "Vitamin C–rich foods should be part of my diet before the scheduled test."
    C. "I will avoid taking aspirin for 7 days before the scheduled test."
    D. "I will continue taking warfarin because it does not impact the test."

56. A patient reports mild breathing difficulty and hoarseness accompanied by frequent urges to clear the throat. Following a laryngoscopy, the patient is diagnosed with dysfunction of the vocal cords. The nurse will:

    A. Encourage taking deep breaths while talking.
    B. Discuss the need for increased rest periods while exercising.
    C. Discuss the need for frequent pulmonary hygiene.
    D. Encourage face-to-face conversations with others.

57. A patient with asthma is scheduled to undergo a pulmonary function test. The nurse should instruct the patient to:

    A. Avoid eating anything for 4 to 8 hours before the test.
    B. Expect a stinging sensation during the test.
    C. Avoid moving or breathing deeply during the test.
    D. Refrain from smoking for 6 to 8 hours before the test.

58. A patient recovering from recent abdominal surgery reports mild difficulty breathing. On auscultation, the nurse hears a light wheezing sound. The nurse should recommend:

    A. Repositioning every 3 to 4 hours.
    B. Avoiding the prone position when lying down.
    C. Frequent coughing.
    D. Complete bed rest for few days.

59. The nurse is caring for a patient who underwent a bowel resection with the creation of an ileostomy 3 days ago. The assessment finding that requires a change to the plan of care is that:

    A. The stoma is dark red and moist.
    B. There is pasty brown stool in the appliance bag.
    C. The peristomal area is red and peeling.
    D. The ostomy appliance bag is deflated.

60. A young adult patient underwent a bowel resection 3 days ago after unsuccessful medical management of Crohn's disease. An ileostomy was created. After the patient's surgery to place the ileostomy, the patient tells the nurse, "I don't want to look at it. Just change the bag, please." An appropriate response by the nurse is:

    A. "I'll do it this time, but you'll have to do it next time."
    B. "Don't worry, it's simple once you get used to it."
    C. "If you change your bag, the doctor will let you go home faster."
    D. "Do you have concerns about changing the bag?"

61. A young adult patient underwent a bowel resection 3 days ago after unsuccessful medical management of Crohn's disease, and an ileostomy was created. The nurse is teaching the patient about stoma and ileostomy care. The nurse knows teaching has been effective when the patient says:

    A. "My stoma should be white and moist."
    B. "I should clean the skin around the stoma."
    C. "I'll change my bag when it is three quarters full."
    D. "I need to be careful when cleaning the inside of my stoma."

62. The provider has progressed the patient admitted for a duodenal ulcer to a full liquid diet. Which selection by the patient requires further education?

    A. Black coffee
    B. Probiotic yogurt shake
    C. Butternut squash soup
    D. Cranberry juice

63. The nurse is preparing a patient with suspected duodenal ulcer for gastroscopy. The patient asks, "Will I be put to sleep during the procedure?" The appropriate nursing response is:

    A. "Yes, you will be given medication so you can sleep during the procedure."
    B. "Don't worry. You won't feel anything during the procedure."
    C. "I'll let the provider know that you have questions about the procedure."
    D. "I'm not sure. The provider will determine the level of anesthesia."

64. The nurse is evaluating a female patient's response to pantoprazole for duodenal ulcer treatment. The laboratory finding that requires follow-up is:

    A. Hemoglobin 13.0 g/dL (8.07 mmol/L).
    B. White blood cell count 15,000 cells/mm³ (1.5 cells 10⁹/L).
    C. Point of care glucose 110 mg/dL (6.11 mmol/L).
    D. Serum magnesium 2.0 mg/dL (0.82 mmol/L).

65. The patient admitted for Addisonian crisis is experiencing peaked T waves on the cardiac monitor. The appropriate nursing action for the nurse to take first is to:

    A. Administer intravenous loop diuretic.
    B. Auscultate the heart sounds.
    C. Give sodium polystyrene sulfonate.
    D. Monitor intake and output.

66. The nurse is caring for a patient admitted for Addisonian crisis. Which assessment finding indicates a therapeutic response to the plan of care?

    A. Blood pressure 106/72 mmHg
    B. Peaked T wave on cardiac monitor
    C. Pink and dry oral mucous membranes
    D. Serum blood glucose 59 mg/dL (3.3 mmol/L)

67. The patient has been prescribed oral prednisone for the management of Addison's disease. Which statement by the patient indicates a need for further teaching?

   A. "I will have to take this medication for the rest of my life."
   B. "At times I should expect to have a fever."
   C. "My blood glucose may need to be monitored."
   D. "The provider may schedule a bone density test."

68. What incident might prompt the nurse to have a swallow evaluation done on a patient with dementia? The patient:

   A. Swallows pills whole but refuses to eat.
   B. Pockets pills in the mouth and coughs after drinking thin liquids.
   C. Needs assistance setting up their food tray and eats very slowly.
   D. Requests to take pills with applesauce and prefers warm drinks.

69. An older adult patient with dementia is confused and keeps exiting the bed, stating that they want to go home. What is the most therapeutic way to communicate with the patient?

   A. Tell the patient they are confused and should stay in bed.
   B. Reorient the patient to the situation and offer to walk with them.
   C. Tell the patient to go to sleep, and then set the bed alarm.
   D. Remind the patient that they have dementia.

70. An older adult patient with dementia has a sudden increase in agitation and impulsiveness. An indwelling Foley catheter is in place due to urinary retention caused by a urinary tract infection (UTI). The nurse notes that there is decreased urine output in the Foley bag. Which intervention would be most appropriate?

   A. Administer olanzapine as needed for increased agitation.
   B. Ensure that the catheter is patent and unobstructed.
   C. Call a rapid response team for change in condition.
   D. Remove the catheter because there is decreased output.

71. A patient with a urinary tract infection (UTI) has been admitted for 24 hours and is receiving broad-spectrum antibiotics. The nurse reviews the morning labs that have resulted. Which lab should the nurse monitor most closely to help the provider select the appropriate medications?

   A. Urine cultures
   B. White blood cell count (WBC)
   C. Hemoglobin
   D. Alanine aminotransferase (ALT) and raised aspartate aminotransferase (AST)

72. An older adult patient is admitted with altered mental status and a urinary tract infection (UTI). The patient has a history of diabetes, kidney stones, and past UTIs. The patient appears confused and agitated. The patient's spouse reports not knowing when the patient last used the bathroom. The patient is now reporting lower abdominal and perineum discomfort and has not urinated since admission. After the patient attempts to urinate, the nurse notes that the agitation is worsening. Upon further evaluation and a postvoid residual bladder scan, it is noted that the patient is retaining 950 mL of urine. What would be the most appropriate nursing intervention?

    A. Insert an indwelling urinary catheter and leave it in place for ease of measuring.
    B. Perform a straight catheterization and reassess for continued urinary retention.
    C. Place an external suction catheter to suction for incontinence.
    D. Have the patient wear an incontinence brief in case they do not reach the bathroom in time.

73. The provider has prescribed ciprofloxacin (Cipro) to a patient with a urinary tract infection (UTI). Which teaching topic should the nurse include in discharge education specific to this medication?

    A. Alert the provider to sudden changes in heart rate.
    B. Know that this medication may turn urine orange.
    C. Discontinue use when you are feeling better.
    D. Separate taking ciprofloxacin and antacids by at least 30 minutes.

74. A patient diagnosed with viral gastroenteritis complains of diarrhea. To improve the diarrhea symptoms, the nurse recommends that the patient:

    A. Adopt a low-fat, low-protein diet.
    B. Increase the amount of fiber and roughage.
    C. Eliminate sugary foods and drinks.
    D. Stop any current vitamin supplements.

75. The nurse is transferring a patient who is 2 days postischemic stroke. The patient has weakness in their left leg, and their left arm is flaccid. How should the nurse care for this patient's arm when transferring?

    A. Allow the patient's arm to dangle freely.
    B. Use the gait belt to secure the patient's arm to their core.
    C. Drape the patient's arm across their body.
    D. Place the patient's arm in a sling.

76. Which statement by a patient with gastroesophageal reflux disease (GERD) indicates an understanding of the disease and its management?

    A. "I should eat more citrus fruits."
    B. "I should avoid caffeinated beverages."
    C. "The provider can prescribe an inhaler for my nighttime cough."
    D. "The ingredients in chocolate can help relieve my symptoms."

77. To prepare a patient on the unit for colostomy care, the nurse will instruct the patient to:

    A. Inspect the stoma daily for discharge and skin integrity.
    B. Remove the pouch before showering.
    C. Perform stoma care when the site is visibly soiled.
    D. Avoid lying on the same side as the stoma site at night.

78. A patient is scheduled to have a colonoscopy at 8 o'clock the next morning. To prepare the patient for the procedure, the nurse will instruct the patient to:

    A. Stop eating and drinking after midnight the night before the procedure.
    B. Avoid eating solid foods at least 24 hours prior to the procedure.
    C. Take prescribed stool softeners 6 hours prior to the procedure.
    D. Increase fluid intake until the time of the procedure to avoid dehydration.

79. What information will the nurse include when teaching the patient techniques to prevent the spread of viral hepatitis?

    A. Do not share personal items, utensils, or tableware.
    B. Handwashing is the only effective measure to prevent spread among household members.
    C. Donate blood only upon completion of treatment for viral hepatitis.
    D. Wear gloves when cooking food at home for others.

80. Which statement by a patient about warning signs of lung cancer indicates the need for additional education?

    A. "Even though my cough is persistent, lack of blood in the sputum means that I do not have cancer."
    B. "When I develop wheezing and chest pain, I should talk to my healthcare provider."
    C. "Frequent blood that I see when coughing into a tissue could be a sign of lung cancer."
    D. "I should watch for changes in my respiratory pattern as a warning sign of lung cancer."

81. Which statement by a patient indicates an understanding of the proper use of an inhaler with a spacer?

    A. "I should inhale the medication after firmly pressing down on the canister."
    B. "I should wait 2 minutes between each puff."
    C. "The whistling sound is an indicator of breathing too rapidly."
    D. "I should clean the spacer when it gets visibly soiled or dirty."

82. What techniques to prevent asthma exacerbation should the nurse teach the patient?

    A. Regular exercise will provide health benefits.
    B. Supplemental oxygen at bedtime will prevent morning attacks.
    C. Use of an albuterol nebulizer every morning will prevent asthma attacks during the day.
    D. Limiting outdoor activities will prevent asthma attacks.

83. To prepare a patient for cardiac catheterization the next morning, the nurse will give the patient which instruction?

   A. "Avoid eating, drinking, and consuming caffeine after midnight."
   B. "Drink plenty of fluids tonight to help prevent dehydration."
   C. "Take a shower tonight to be clean for the procedure."
   D. "Tell the provider about any metal objects in your body."

84. When educating a patient with a newly placed chest tube and attached collection unit, the nurse will instruct the patient to:

   A. Keep all tubing free of kinks to prevent occlusions.
   B. Put the collection unit on a side table during mealtimes.
   C. Expect to hear vigorous bubbling within the collection unit.
   D. Reposition in bed as desired regardless of placement of the collection unit.

85. What information will be included when educating a patient on recognizing the differences between signs of left-sided and right-sided heart failure?

   A. Right-sided heart failure is characterized by weak peripheral pulses.
   B. Left-sided heart failure is characterized by unexpected weight gain.
   C. Right-sided heart failure is characterized by neck vein distention.
   D. Left-sided heart failure is characterized by edema in the lower extremities.

86. A patient asks the nurse about warning signs of leukemia. The nurse reviews acute signs, including:

   A. Increased thirst during the day.
   B. Daytime somnolence.
   C. Excessive bruising.
   D. Significant reduction in heart rate.

87. The nurse is caring for a patient who underwent kidney transplant 3 months ago. Which of the following findings would the nurse identify as being the most indicative of the acute phase of transplant rejection?

   A. Drop in hemoglobin level
   B. Increased creatinine level
   C. Elevated sedimentary rate
   D. Presence of glucosuria

88. To prepare a patient for management of diabetes by insulin at home, the nurse will instruct the patient to:

   A. Dose sliding-scale insulin throughout the day based on the morning glucose.
   B. Check their blood sugar any time they notice that they do not feel well.
   C. Avoid eating meals late in the evening and eliminate bedtime snacks.
   D. Carry all insulins on their person at all times to be used as needed.

89. The patient is diagnosed with Cushing's disease. The nurse will instruct the patient to:

    A. Perform frequent handwashing.
    B. Avoid physical activity.
    C. Follow a low-protein diet.
    D. Avoid outdoor activities.

90. The patient is diagnosed with syndrome of inappropriate antidiuretic hormone (SIADH). The nurse will instruct the patient to:

    A. Limit the amount of free water in the diet to 1 L.
    B. Drink plenty of fluids throughout the day.
    C. Avoid contact sports and labor-intensive activities.
    D. Obtain weight daily and report more than 2-lb weight gain to the provider.

91. Which statement by a patient with a urinary catheter indicates an understanding of its function?

    A. "The balloon at the catheter tip stops the catheter from becoming dislodged."
    B. "I should pull on the catheter gently to be sure it has not migrated from the bladder."
    C. "Drinking plenty of fluids during the day will help to maintain catheter patency."
    D. "I should let air out of the urine container to maintain catheter patency."

92. The nurse is caring for a patient who sustained a tibia fracture 2 days ago secondary to a crush injury. Swelling has been present in the area since the injury. Which of the following should be urgently reported to the provider?

    A. Sudden, severe pain that is not controlled with pain medications
    B. Pain with abduction and adduction of the affected leg
    C. Swelling that is not resolved when the leg is evaluated
    D. Persistent bruising that extends from the patella to the ankle

93. To prepare a patient on the unit for management of urinary incontinence upon discharge, the nurse will instruct the patient to:

    A. Perform pelvic floor muscle exercises every day.
    B. Change incontinence pads one to two times per day.
    C. Drink carbonated beverages to facilitate urination.
    D. Perform self-catheterization when there is abdominal pressure.

94. Which statement is true about delirium?

    A. It develops over hours to days.
    B. It is often caused by a single factor.
    C. Thinking is intact but fatigue is present.
    D. It has a duration of several years.

95. The nurse is caring for a patient with myasthenia gravis who is receiving treatment with neostigmine. Which assessment finding would alert the nurse that the patient may be experiencing a cholinergic crisis?

    A. Abdominal pain
    B. Respiratory distress
    C. Tachycardia
    D. Dilated pupils

96. The nurse is admitting a patient diagnosed with tetanus. Which action should the nurse take initially?

    A. Assess respiratory status.
    B. Administer antibiotics.
    C. Implement seizure precautions.
    D. Provide wound care.

97. Which type of tube would the nurse recommend to the provider for a patient who needs short-term gastric decompression?

    A. Nasogastric
    B. Nasoduodenal
    C. Gastrostomy
    D. Jejunostomy

98. The nurse is caring for an adult patient admitted for an upper gastrointestinal (GI) bleed who has a long history of alcohol misuse. Which symptom would suggest that the GI bleed may be due to a Mallory–Weiss tear?

    A. Currant jelly stools
    B. Microcytic anemia
    C. Recent history of vomiting
    D. Increased urine output

99. Which medication would the nurse anticipate administering to form a protective barrier against acid for a patient with peptic ulcer disease?

    A. Sucralfate (Carafate)
    B. Metoclopramide (Reglan)
    C. Aluminum hydroxide, magnesium hydroxide (Maalox)
    D. Lansoprazole (Prevacid)

100. A patient presents to the ED with an occult gastrointestinal (GI) bleed. Which action should the nurse take first?

    A. Place two large-bore intravenous lines.
    B. Measure the urine output.
    C. Insert a nasogastric (NG) tube.
    D. Obtain laboratory specimens.

101. The nurse is preparing to suction a patient with a tracheostomy. Which action is proper suctioning procedure?

    A. Insert the catheter with continuous suction on.
    B. Wait at least 30 seconds after each suctioning pass.
    C. Advance the catheter until it touches the carina.
    D. Complete the procedure using clean technique.

102. The nurse is caring for a patient who will undergo an esophagogastroduodenoscopy (EGD). Which intervention should be included in the patient's plan of care?

    A. Prepare the patient for general anesthesia.
    B. Keep the patient on nothing-by-mouth (NPO) status for 4 hours before the procedure.
    C. Check the patient's temperature every 15 to 30 minutes for 1 to 2 hours post procedure.
    D. Keep the patient NPO after the procedure until bowel sounds return.

103. Which intervention is appropriate for a patient being admitted to the medical–surgical unit with a diagnosis of tuberculosis?

    A. Place the patient in a positive-pressure room.
    B. Never transport the patient within the hospital.
    C. Perform a Mantoux test.
    D. Allow only fit-tested employees to care for the patient.

104. The nurse is caring for a patient with a chest tube placed secondary to a pneumothorax. The chest tube is connected to a disposable chest drainage unit. Which intervention represents appropriate care for this patient?

    A. Empty the drainage unit when full.
    B. Redress the insertion site with a vented dressing.
    C. Ensure there is constant bubbling in the drainage unit's water-seal chamber.
    D. Place the wall suction regulator on continuous suction.

105. The nurse is caring for a patient who is admitted with multiple rib fractures. Which action by the nurse would be most appropriate for this patient?

    A. Apply a thoracic binder.
    B. Place the patient in the Trendelenburg position.
    C. Promote deep breathing and coughing.
    D. Avoid administering opioid pain medications.

106. The nurse is caring for a patient with a tracheostomy tube that becomes dislodged. Which action should the nurse take first?

    A. Call for help.
    B. Assess the patient's level of consciousness.
    C. Retrieve the safety kit with obturator and spare tube.
    D. Provide supplemental oxygen.

107. Which intervention is appropriate nursing care for a patient who has returned to the medical–surgical unit after permanent pacemaker placement?

    A. Encourage active range of motion on the operative side.
    B. Keep the patient on bed rest for at least 3 days.
    C. Adjust the pacemaker's sensitivity as needed for capture.
    D. Monitor the patient's temperature.

108. The nurse is caring for a patient admitted with a diagnosis of pulmonary embolism (PE). Which intervention should the nurse complete first?

    A. Assess cardiopulmonary status.
    B. Insert a peripheral intravenous line.
    C. Initiate fall precautions.
    D. Place the patient in semi-Fowler's to promote breathing.

109. The nurse is caring for a patient who is diagnosed with a venous thromboembolism (VTE) and taking warfarin (Coumadin) for anticoagulation. Which intervention represents appropriate nursing care?

    A. Massage the affected extremity.
    B. Promote early ambulation of the patient.
    C. Monitor partial thromboplastin time (PTT) for effectiveness of warfarin.
    D. Promote intake of green, leafy vegetables.

110. The nurse is caring for a patient with a history of implantable cardioverter-defibrillator (ICD) placement. The patient reports that the device delivered a single shock. Which action should the nurse take first?

    A. Check the patient's vital signs.
    B. Notify the provider.
    C. Assure the patient that nothing is wrong.
    D. Obtain an EKG.

111. Which action should the nurse include in the immediate plan of care for a patient newly admitted for a hypertensive emergency?

    A. Lower the patient's blood pressure as quickly as possible.
    B. Use the mean arterial pressure (MAP) to guide and evaluate treatment.
    C. Encourage ambulation of the patient.
    D. Administer oral antihypertensives to the patient.

112. The nurse is caring for a patient diagnosed with acute coronary syndrome. Which intervention is the priority action?

    A. Place the patient on supplemental oxygen.
    B. Administer nitroglycerin to the patient.
    C. Direct the patient to chew a 325-mg aspirin.
    D. Slowly push morphine intravenously.

113. A nurse is caring for a patient diagnosed with gout who is prescribed allopurinol (Zyloprim). Which signs and symptoms would indicate that the patient may be experiencing Stevens–Johnson syndrome?

    A. A rash develops immediately following administration of the drug.
    B. Painless mucosal lesions appear on the palms, soles, and trunk.
    C. Systemic symptoms, such as fever, cough, and nausea, develop.
    D. Vesicles occur distributed linearly along a dermatome.

114. The nurse is caring for a patient with Alzheimer's disease. Which action by the nurse would represent appropriate care of the patient?

    A. If chewing and swallowing is problematic, offer a thin, liquid diet.
    B. Monitor for behavior changes as a manifestation of pain.
    C. Limit liquids to mealtimes only.
    D. Correct misstatements or faulty memories.

115. Which symptoms are the most common manifestation of gastrointestinal disease?

    A. Nausea and vomiting
    B. Anorexia
    C. Heartburn
    D. Diarrhea

116. The nurse is caring for a patient who is experiencing dumping syndrome following gastrectomy. Which action by the nurse represents appropriate care of this patient?

    A. Divide meals into six small feedings.
    B. Give additional fluids with meals.
    C. Offer concentrated sweets like honey or jelly.
    D. Encourage foods high in insoluble fiber.

117. The nurse is caring for a patient who presents with abdominal cramping and diarrhea. The patient reports that they prepared chicken for dinner last night but stopped eating it partway through upon noticing that the chicken was pink in the middle. Which of the following is the most likely cause of the patient's acute infectious diarrhea?

    A. *Clostridium difficile*
    B. *Giardia lamblia*
    C. *Entamoeba histolytica*
    D. *Campylobacter jejuni*

118. The nurse is caring for a patient with chronic hepatitis. Which assessment finding would alert the nurse that the patient may be experiencing fulminant hepatic failure?

    A. Azotemia
    B. Jaundice
    C. Alanine transaminase (ALT)/aspartate transaminase (AST) elevations
    D. Hepatomegaly

119. Which assessment finding is consistent with a patient experiencing atelectasis?

    A. Decreased or absent breath sounds
    B. Resonance to percussion over the lungs
    C. Wheezes upon auscultation
    D. Accentuation of pulmonic heart sound

120. Which term refers to lung diseases caused by inhalation and retention of mineral or metal dust particles?

    A. Pneumoconiosis
    B. Sarcoidosis
    C. Tuberculosis
    D. Pleurisy

121. Assistive personnel report that the patient is experiencing dyspnea. Which action should the nurse first take to assess for a tension pneumothorax?

    A. Auscultate lung sounds.
    B. Check pulse oximetry levels.
    C. Check respiratory rate.
    D. Assess the skin for diaphoresis.

122. A patient is admitted to the medical–surgical unit with pneumonia. Which observation by the nurse would indicate that the patient is worsening?

    A. The provider has changed the antibiotic route to oral.
    B. The patient has not responded to antibiotic therapy within 12 hours.
    C. The patient continues to be febrile after 24 hours.
    D. The patient's arterial blood gas shows hypercapnia after 72 hours.

123. The nurse is caring for a young adult patient diagnosed with community-acquired pneumonia (CAP) who is otherwise healthy. Which action by the nurse would represent appropriate care of this patient?

    A. Limiting the intake of oral fluids during the day
    B. Placing the patient in the supine position at bedtime
    C. Drawing blood cultures from the existing intravenous (IV) sites
    D. Ambulating in the hall with the medical assistant

124. After a few days of treatment for tuberculosis, the patient develops an orange discoloration of bodily fluids. Which medication that the patient recently received may be a contributing factor?

    A. Isoniazid
    B. Rifampin
    C. Pyrazinamide
    D. Ethambutol

125. The nurse is caring for a patient with hypertension who is taking carvedilol (Coreg). Which symptom would indicate that the patient may be experiencing a side effect of the medication?

    A. Dizziness on standing
    B. Dry cough
    C. Bronchospasm
    D. Tachycardia

126. Which symptom is specific to right-sided heart failure?

    A. Abdominal ascites
    B. Left ventricular hypertrophy
    C. Fluid accumulation in the lungs
    D. Poor exercise tolerance

127. The nurse is caring for a patient with coronary artery disease. Which assessment finding requires the nurse's immediate action?

    A. Proteinuria
    B. Intermittent claudication
    C. Absent dorsalis pedis pulses
    D. Increased afterload

128. The nurse is caring for a patient with iron-deficiency anemia who is receiving sodium ferrous gluconate intravenously. Which lab value should the nurse monitor to assess for response to therapy?

    A. Hemoglobin (Hgb)
    B. Mean corpuscular volume (MCV)
    C. Serum ferritin
    D. Total iron-binding capacity (TIBC)

129. Which type of anemia is classified as microcytic and hypochromic?

    A. Iron-deficiency anemia
    B. Vitamin B12 deficiency
    C. Aplastic anemia
    D. Sickle cell anemia

130. The nurse is caring for a patient with sickle cell disease (SCD) who reports fatigue and malaise. Which assessment finding requires the nurse's immediate attention?

    A. Unchanged anemia on complete blood count
    B. Persistent low-grade fever
    C. Chronic, intermittent joint pain
    D. Normal creatinine level

131. The nurse is assessing the abdomen of a patient who reports stomach pain. Which action will the nurse take first?

    A. Percuss
    B. Inspect
    C. Palpate
    D. Auscultate

132. The nurse is monitoring a patient who receives bolus enteral feedings through a nasogastric (NG) tube. Before administering a feeding, the nurse will measure the gastric residual to:

    A. Confirm the placement of the NG tube.
    B. Remove gastric acid that might cause irritation.
    C. Determine the patient's electrolyte balance.
    D. Identify delayed gastric emptying.

133. The nurse is teaching the partner of a patient with dysphagia how to feed them to prevent aspiration. Which statement by the partner shows that the teaching was effective?

    A. "My partner will be in the supine position."
    B. "My partner will put the food in the center their mouth when eating."
    C. "My partner will tilt their head forward when swallowing."
    D. "My partner will lie down immediately after eating to rest."

134. Which action will the nurse take first when caring for a patient with gastrointestinal bleeding?

    A. Obtain vital signs.
    B. Administer pain medication.
    C. Perform fecal occult blood testing.
    D. Prepare the patient for upper gastrointestinal series.

135. The nurse is caring for a patient with a wound who needs to increase protein intake. Which food will the nurse recommend as the best source of protein?

    A. One cup of whole milk
    B. One whole egg
    C. One half-cup of cottage cheese
    D. One half of a chicken breast

136. The nurse is preparing for admission of a patient with active pulmonary tuberculosis (TB). Which action will the healthcare team take?

    A. Wear surgical masks when caring for the patient.
    B. Educate the patient's roommate on airborne precautions.
    C. Assign the patient to a positive-pressure room.
    D. Have the patient wear a mask during transport.

137. The nurse is treating a patient during end-of-life care. The patient has been prescribed morphine. When creating a plan of care, the nurse will educate the patient to:

    A. Stop the medication if it causes pruritus.
    B. Maintain normal activities while taking medication.
    C. Actively cough to prevent secretion buildup.
    D. Stop the medication if constipation occurs.

138. Which action will the nurse take when suctioning a patient with a tracheostomy?

    A. Apply suctioning while advancing the suction catheter.
    B. Preoxygenate the patient with 100% oxygen.
    C. Limit the suction pass to 30 seconds.
    D. Suction the patient as many times as needed.

139. The nurse alerts the emergency response team upon witnessing a patient experiencing symptomatic bradycardia. The nurse anticipates that the emergency response team will administer:

    A. Metoprolol.
    B. Diltiazem.
    C. Adenosine.
    D. Atropine.

140. A patient taking diltiazem and digoxin for atrial fibrillation reports abdominal cramping and nausea. For which additional cue would the nurse evaluate when considering toxicity?

    A. Increased appetite
    B. Constipation
    C. Confusion
    D. Increased energy

141. The nurse is monitoring an older patient with peripheral vascular disease (PVD) who reports difficulty sleeping because of cold feet. Which intervention will best help address the patient's concern?

    A. Place nonslip socks on the patient's feet.
    B. Place a heating pad under the patient's feet.
    C. Provide warm beverages to the patient.
    D. Use lanolin on the patient's feet.

142. The nurse is planning care for a patient who is to receive packed red blood cells. Transfusion of a bag should be completed within how many hours?

    A. 4
    B. 5
    C. 6
    D. 7

143. The nurse is providing education to a patient who has diabetes mellitus and receives neutral protamine Hagedorn (NPH) insulin every morning with meals. Which information will the nurse include?

    A. Mix the NPH solution vigorously before using.
    B. Throw away NPH solution if it is cloudy.
    C. Put unused NPH solutions in the freezer.
    D. Be aware that NPH is expected to peak in 4 to 12 hours.

144. The nurse is assessing a postoperative patient who has anemia due to excessive blood loss after surgery. Which finding will the nurse expect?

    A. Increased appetite
    B. Bradycardia
    C. Hypertension
    D. Lethargy

145. When teaching patients how to monitor for hypoglycemia, which sign would be included?

    A. Increased urination
    B. Tremors
    C. Acetone-smelling breath
    D. Bradycardia

146. The nurse is educating a patient with diabetes about preventing diabetic ketoacidosis (DKA) during an illness. Which instructions will the nurse include in the education?

    A. Decrease fluid intake.
    B. Check blood glucose every 6 hours.
    C. Stop taking insulin for the duration of the illness.
    D. Check urine for ketones every 4 hours.

147. A patient with diabetes mellitus was given short-acting regular insulin via a sliding scale at 9:00 a.m. The nurse will ensure that the patient receives breakfast at which time?

    A. 9:15 a.m.
    B. 9:30 a.m.
    C. 10:15 a.m.
    D. 10:30 a.m.

CASE STUDY

A patient experiencing sickle cell crisis has been admitted. Vital signs are as follows: temperature 98.9°F (37.2°C); pulse 118 beats/min; respiration rate 22 breaths/min; blood pressure 90/47 mmHg; oxygen saturation 80% on room air. The patient states, "I feel dizzy when walking or standing." The patient reports pain of 9/10 in the flank area and back. The patient has been able to urinate, but the urine appears very concentrated.

Lab Test	Value
White blood cell count (WBC)	13,000/µL (13 × 10⁹/L)
Red blood cell count (RBC)	4 million cells/µL (4 × 10¹²/L)
Hemoglobin	7.2 g/dL (4.47 mmol/L)
Lactic acid	1.5 mg/dL (0.1665 mmol/L)
Creatinine	1.75 mg/dL (154.74 µmol/L)
Partial pressure of oxygen (PaO₂)	80 mmHg (10.6 kPa)
Partial pressure of carbon dioxide (PaCO₂)	34 mmHg (4.53 kPa)

148. The priority intervention, given the vital signs and laboratory values of this patient, is to:

    A. Administer pain medication based on the 9/10 rating.
    B. Place nasal cannula to provide supplemental oxygen.
    C. Start peripheral intravenous (IV) line to deliver a bolus of normal saline.
    D. Ask the patient when their last bowel movement was.

149. Which laboratory value would alert the nurse that acute kidney injury (AKI) is occurring?

    A. Red blood cells (RBC) of 4 million cells/µL (4 × 10¹²/L)
    B. White blood cells (WBC) of 13,000/µL (13 × 10⁹/L)
    C. Hemoglobin of 7.2 g/dL (4.47 mmol/L)
    D. Creatinine of 1.75 mg/dL (154.74 µmol/L)

150. While continuing to assess the patient, the set of objective data that would alert the nurse to call the provider and anticipate a possible blood transfusion is:

    A. Blood pressure of 110/64 mmHg and temperature of 98.9°F (37.2°C).
    B. Respiratory rate of 18 breaths/min at rest and oxygen saturation of 93% on 4 LPM (liters per minute) per nasal cannula.
    C. Pale skin and hemoglobin level of 6.5 g/dL (4.03 mmol/L).
    D. Urine output above 30 mL/hr and creatinine of 1.2 mg/dL (106.1 µmol/L).

MSNCB Certification Practice Exam: Answers

1. D) Oliguric
The phases of AKI are onset, oliguric, diuretic, and recovery. Urine output of less than 400 mL in 24 hours indicates that the patient is in the oliguric phase. During onset, output is less than 0.5 mL/kg/hr. In the diuretic phase, daily urine output is 1 to 2 L. The recovery phase can take several months but indicates that laboratory values are stabilizing.

2. C) Ataxic.
Ataxic gait is caused by a neurogenic disorder, such as spinal cord lesions, and causes a staggering, uncoordinated gait with a sway. Festinating gait is caused by a neurogenic disorder such as Parkinson's disease; the patient walks with short, shuffling steps, and the patient's neck, trunk, and knees flex while the body is rigid. Spastic gait is a result of a neurogenic disorder such as cerebral palsy; it involves stiffness in one or both legs that causes the affected leg to swing outward and drag the foot forward with each step. Steppage gait is caused by a neurogenic disorder such as peroneal nerve injury; increased hip and knee flexion are needed to clear the foot from the floor, and foot drop is evident.

3. C) Hematuria
Hematuria can be caused by ruptured cysts in the kidneys. Among the first symptoms of PKD are pain and hypertension. Kidneys can be palpable on examination due to enlargement from cysts.

4. B) Provide family photos and familiar objects to the patient.
Family photos and familiar objects are memory triggers that can help with a patient's agitation and confusion. Patients with Alzheimer's disease should not be encouraged to go for a ride with a family member unless they show feelings of comfort around that person; otherwise, this could cause more stress and confusion. Scheduled activities have been found to be more beneficial for patients with Alzheimer's disease than allowing them to follow their own schedule. Talking about or to the patient as if they were a child is not an effective or appropriate way to manage the stress or confusion of the patient.

5. B) Write down the order and then read it back to the provider.
When receiving a telephone or other verbal order from a provider, the nurse should write down the order and then read back the complete order to the provider to verify its accuracy. Immediately carrying out the order and documenting the order without verification are both unsafe practices because they present the risk of inappropriate interventions. Although receiving written orders is preferable to receiving telephone orders, the latter is sometimes necessary.

6. B) Depressed thoughts

Isotretinoin is thought to increase the risk of suicidal ideation in a small number of patients. A patient reporting depressed thoughts should be evaluated immediately for risk of self-harm. Pruritus, increased sensitivity to sunlight (with increased potential for sunburn), and stomach upset are less serious side effects. Although the patient should feel free to contact the provider if they have questions about these effects, there is no need for urgent intervention.

7. A) Peer-reviewed journals.

Reliable sources include peer-reviewed journals, systematic reviews, pre-appraised literature, and practice guidelines. Online discussion groups and nursing textbooks are too general and are not reliable sources. Research articles in prepublication form may not have been properly vetted or peer reviewed.

8. A) Do not assume responsibility for disclosure before speaking to the provider.

Following serious unanticipated outcomes, including those clearly caused by system failures, the patient, and the family if necessary, should receive timely, transparent, and clear communication concerning what is known about the event. Information should be provided to the patient and the family once all information has been received and should be communicated by the appropriate member of the healthcare team. The provider is generally responsible for discussing surgical outcomes with the patient and/or the family. Other agency representatives may be involved in the disclosure process, including administrators, risk managers, and attorneys. The nurse should not disclose or deny any information at this time. The nurse should relay any patient or family concerns to the provider to ensure that they are addressed. The role of the hospital ombuds is to address patient or family complaints, which is not the current situation. Should the patient or family have a concern or complaint after discussing the situation, the ombuds may become involved; they are not the initial point of contact in this situation.

9. C) Performing consistent hand hygiene.

Because nearly all nursing care involves physical contact with patients and physical objects, complying with either the current Centers for Disease Control and Prevention hand-hygiene guidelines or the current World Health Organization hand-hygiene guidelines is the most effective way to reduce the risk of healthcare-associated infections. Providing annual influenza vaccinations is effective in reducing transmission of influenza but does not impact other potential sources of infection. Wearing a mask during patient care is required when there is a risk of airborne transmission, but this is a subset of nursing care. Up-to-date employee health records can help track immunization status but are otherwise limited in their ability to help control infection risk.

10. B) Urinate after sexual intercourse.

Urinating after sexual intercourse helps to clear secretions that may have reached the urethra, thus reducing the risk for developing a UTI. Voiding regularly, such as every 3 to 4 hours, during the day is recommended, but the patient should not be advised to frequently strain or force themselves to urinate. The nurse should emphasize the importance of taking the full course of antibiotics, even if symptoms improve, to ensure complete treatment of the infection. Fluids will increase frequency of urination but will also dilute the urine, making the bladder less irritable.

11. D) Hyperventilation
In DKA, the patient has Kussmaul respirations, a type of hyperventilation. The patient will usually have mild hyponatremia, not hypernatremia. Normal serum potassium is unlikely; the patient will have hyperkalemia initially, and then hypokalemia. Slightly rapid respirations would be common in hyperosmolar hyperglycemic nonketotic syndrome, another acute complication of diabetes.

12. D) Adopting a low-calcium diet.
Patients with calcium renal calculi (kidney stones) may have to make dietary modifications to prevent the formation of future stones. A low-calcium diet is recommended for patients with a history of calcium oxalate calculi to limit the amount of calcium available for stone production. Increased intake of high-fiber foods helps bind calcium and reduces the risk of stones. Although high consumption of animal protein is thought to contribute to calculi development, there is no reason to limit overall protein intake as long as a significant portion consists of plant protein. Sodium intake does not have a major impact on stone formation. Also, the nurse should exercise caution before advising any patient to increase sodium intake due to its significant effects on chronic medical conditions such as hypertension.

13. D) Administer a simple carbohydrate to the patient.
Hypoglycemia is a concerning finding that requires immediate intervention. Because the patient is experiencing signs and symptoms of hypoglycemia, the initial action would be to administer a simple carbohydrate to raise the blood glucose level. Simple carbohydrates are recommended because they break down quickly for faster glucose availability. The patient's blood sugar should be checked after a carbohydrate is administered to ensure that the blood glucose level is going up; this is usually done 15 to 30 minutes after carbohydrate administration. The administration time may need to be altered if the patient is having multiple hypoglycemic episodes, but this would be assessed after the low glucose was addressed. Similarly, reinforcing education on proper diet should take place after addressing this hypoglycemic episode.

14. C) Low free T3.
Weight gain, fatigue, impaired memory, and a slow pulse rate, along with decreased levels of free T3 (triiodothyronine) and free T4 (thyroxine), indicate hypothyroidism. TSH (thyroid-stimulating hormone) will be high. The total T4 is expected to be low.

15. D) Hyponatremia
The clinical picture of Addison's disease includes muscle weakness, anorexia, darkening of the skin, and polydipsia. Polydipsia is present secondary to a low sodium level that is commonly seen with the condition. Other expected lab values include hyperkalemia, hypoglycemia, and a low cortisol level.

16. C) Psoriasis.
Psoriasis, a chronic skin disorder with an unknown cause, can result in thick, reddened papules or plaques covered by silver-white scales. Scabies are mites that burrow under the skin, generally between the webbing of the fingers and toes. They create tracks of small blisters or bumps on the skin. Seborrhea (also known as *cradle cap*) is a chronic inflammatory dermatitis that typically affects the scalp. Squamous cell carcinoma appears as a red, crusted, scaly patch on the skin; a raised growth with a depressed center; or a firm, red-black nodule.

17. D) Renal sonography.

The most helpful diagnostic tool for polycystic kidney disease is renal sonography, which can assess for the presence and size of renal cysts. A CT scan of the abdomen could identify renal cysts, but not to the degree that a direct visualization of the kidneys via ultrasound would provide. Additionally, a CT scan would result in unnecessary radiation exposure. Laboratory tests, such as hemoglobin A1C, CBC, and BMP are part of the general evaluation but are not specific to the diagnosis of polycystic kidney disease.

18. B) Restricted mobility

Urinary incontinence occurs when the bladder pressure exceeds the urethral closure pressure. Anything that interferes with bladder or urethral sphincter control can result in incontinence. Using the acronym DRIP, the causes can include *D:* delirium, dehydration, depression; *R:* restricted mobility, rectal impaction; *I:* infection, inflammation, impaction; and *P:* polyuria, polypharmacy. The presence of dizziness, pruritis, and petechiae do not indicate risk for incontinence.

19. A) "I'm really bad about staying hydrated."

Kidney stones can be caused by a buildup of minerals in the urine. Dehydration can cause these minerals to collect and form a stone. Increased stress and exercise are not considered risk factors for renal calculi formation. Unfortified orange juice does not contain ingredients that would increase the risk of renal calculi.

20. D) Limiting dietary protein intake.

When a kidney injury and/or renal impairment is present, the intake of dietary protein should be limited. The byproduct of protein breakdown is more difficult for the kidneys to eliminate when they are impaired. Rest is recommended until the signs of glomerular inflammation (proteinuria, hematuria) and hypertension subside. Restricted sodium and fluid intake can help reduce edema. Although most cases of poststreptococcal glomerulonephritis resolve over time with little to no residual effects, a small proportion of patients will develop long-term renal effects. At this time, there is nothing to indicate dialysis is needed.

21. D) Sepsis.

Sepsis can lead to vascular collapse, which can cause the organs to receive inadequate perfusion. This can lead to prerenal failure. Renal carcinoma and aminoglycoside toxicity are renal causes, and ureterolithiasis is a postrenal cause.

22. B) Promote self-care independence.

An overall goal associated with OA treatment includes implementing measures that promote the highest degree of independent functioning. The ability to independently perform self-care tasks is an appropriate and obtainable goal for most patients with OA as it aims to help the patient meet their most basic needs. The joint damage and bony abnormalities that result from the condition are considered permanent; the goal is to prevent further damage, not reverse it. Medications are prescribed to minimize pain, which leads to increased activity, but the prescribed medications will not eliminate all pain because this is a chronic condition.

23. D) Cardiac catheterization

Pulmonary hypertension is diagnosed by measuring a patient's pulmonary artery pressure, cardiac output, and pulmonary vascular resistance. A right-sided cardiac catheterization is an invasive procedure that allows for direct measurement of pressures within the heart, allowing for accurate diagnosis. The outcomes produced by the high pressures associated with pulmonary hypertension can be seen on an EKG, chest x-ray, and CT scan, but these tests cannot measure pressures and thus do not provide the information needed to make the diagnosis.

24. C) Vitiligo

Vitiligo is a complete absence of melanin (pigment) resulting in chalky-white patches. Alopecia is loss of hair (localized or general). Telangiectasia involves visibly dilated, superficial, cutaneous small blood vessels, commonly found on the face and thighs. Lichenification is thickening of the skin with accentuated normal skin markings.

25. B) "I know that the medication should be kept refrigerated at all times."

Although nitroglycerin requires protection from light and high heat, storing the medication in the refrigerator is unnecessary. Also, the patient should carry the medication with them at all times; placing the medication in the refrigerator separates the patient from the medication. It is appropriate to repeat the dose every 5 minutes for a maximum of three times. Nitroglycerin tablets are stored in light-resistant bottles with metal caps and should be replaced every 6 months.

26. A) Epinephrine 1:1,000, 0.3 mL to 0.5 mL intramuscularly (IM) or intravenously (IV).

Epinephrine should be administered immediately to any patient who is experiencing the life-threatening signs and symptoms of anaphylaxis. The proper dose would be epinephrine 1:1,000 aqueous solution, 0.3 to 0.5 mL given subcutaneously every 20 to 30 minutes for up to three doses, or 5 mL of a 1:10,000 solution given by slow IV infusion every 5 to 10 minutes as needed. Diphenhydramine, prednisone, and famotidine are also given to help counter histamine-mediated reactions, but these medications are given after epinephrine due to its faster onset.

27. B) Provide monitoring for dysrhythmias and decompensation.

The nurse should monitor the patient for the dysrhythmias and decompensation that can occur secondary to thyrotoxicosis. Medications that decrease (not increase) thyroid hormone production would be administered. Multiple doses of dexamethasone would be given at 1 to 2 mg every 6 hours for thyroid storm.

28. A) "Check your blood sugar at least every 3 to 4 hours."

Blood sugar levels may continue to fluctuate after discharge, so the patient should check their blood sugar several times throughout the day as well as any time they feel symptoms of hyperglycemia or hypoglycemia. Fluids should not be restricted but encouraged to prevent dehydration and replace volume that was lost due to the diabetic ketoacidosis. The patient should follow their prescribed diet; there is no need to increase fiber content at this time. Any alteration in temperature would be considered abnormal because temperature changes are not associated with diabetic ketoacidosis.

29. D) Embolic stroke

Most emboli originate in the endocardial layer of the heart when plaque breaks off from the endocardium and enters circulation. The embolus travels up to the cerebral circulation and lodges where a vessel narrows or splits. Heart conditions, such as atrial fibrillation, account for most embolic ischemic strokes. No other neurologic conditions, such as traumatic injury or Parkinson's disease, correlate with atrial fibrillation. Hemorrhagic stroke results from bleeding in the brain.

30. C) Pain in the arm worsens when the arm is positioned at the level of the shoulder.

The pain that is associated with compartment syndrome is primarily due to ischemia. Elevating the limb above the level of the heart decreases circulation, which worsens ischemia and intensifies pain. Pain caused by placing the arm in a dependent position is consistent with generalized swelling or impingement syndrome. Full flexion or extension of the arm is most likely to result in increased, not resolved, pain. Pain radiating to the scapula would not be consistent with compartment syndrome, and the clinical pictures does not suggest direct involvement of the scapula.

31. C) Chronic sun exposure.

Sun exposure is the most common cause of basal cell carcinoma. Burns, immunosuppression, and radiation exposure are less common causes.

32. B) Educate the patient on the dietary approaches to stop hypertension (DASH) diet and the importance of regular exercise.

Dietary modifications and physical exercise support optimal outcomes in the management of hypertension. Although it would be important for the patient to follow up with their primary care provider, a diagnosis of hypertension does not warrant immediate follow-up upon every elevated reading at home. The patient should be given parameters for reporting elevated blood pressure readings. Salt reduction is recommended; however, there is no indication that fluid intake should be limited. Fluid restrictions are recommended for cardiac conditions such as congestive heart failure. An urgent cardiology referral would be indicated if the patient's hypertension was severe and unable to be controlled with first-line medications.

33. D) Hemophilia

Hemophilia is an X-linked recessive genetic disorder caused by a defective or deficient clotting factor. Thrombocytopenia is a disorder defined by a low level of circulating platelets. Thalassemia is an anemia characterized by red blood cell (RBC) destruction beyond the bone marrow's ability to produce these cells. Sickle cell anemia is a genetic disorder that causes malformation of RBCs.

34. A) Recheck the blood pressure manually in both arms.

Before acting on the blood pressure reading, the nurse should recheck the blood pressure to determine the accuracy of the reading. Assessing for heart disease would not be an immediate intervention and would be conducted later, after the patient's blood pressure has been rechecked. If the reported blood pressure is accurate, it warrants immediate intervention, so waiting 4 hours to recheck the blood pressure would be unsafe and places the patient at risk for complications associated with an extremely high blood pressure. No medication should be administered until the blood pressure is confirmed; there is no indication that the elevated blood pressure is being caused by pain.

35. A) Contact the medical provider and clarify the orders.

Corticosteroids will raise blood sugar levels and will require close monitoring while the patient is receiving therapy. Therefore, the first action would be to clarify orders with the medical provider to ensure the order is correct. By contacting the provider, the nurse can confirm the ordered medication and obtain orders for appropriate blood sugar monitoring. At times, alternative medications, such as a steroid inhaler, can be used that have less of an effect on blood sugar levels. The home regimen might not be sufficient to address elevated blood sugars that result from illness and corticosteroid therapy. Oral corticosteroids do not have to be taken with food, and adding an unnecessary snack will raise blood sugar levels further. The nurse should clarify the blood sugar check schedule during the initial contact with the provider; the nurse should not independently initiate checks every 2 hours.

36. D) Peak effects are seen within 2 to 3 hours.

It is important to differentiate the action of immediate-release metformin from that of extended-release metformin. A dose of immediate-release metformin peaks in 2 to 3 hours. It also has a plasma half-life of 4 to 9 hours, and optimal effects are seen within days, up to 2 weeks. Metformin is primarily excreted by the kidneys, not the liver.

37. D) Fluid and electrolyte balance

Hyperaldosteronism involves excessive aldosterone secretion that affects the fluid and electrolyte balance, including sodium retention and potassium excretion. Excretion of urinary waste, blood perfusion to the lungs, and altered gastrointestinal function are not affected by hyperaldosteronism.

38. A) Educate the patient on the vaccine, including desired outcomes and possible side effects.

The first step in administering any medication, especially a vaccine, is to educate the patient. The patient should be educated regarding all aspects of the vaccine before providing consent; the associated vaccine education document should also be provided. There is no guarantee the patient will develop a fever, so there is no need to premedicate the patient. Mild erythema and soreness may be seen for 2 to 3 days after administration of the vaccine. However, swelling, pain, and discoloration are red flags that the patient should report to the healthcare provider. There is no benefit to repeating the influenza vaccine if the patient has an acute episode of influenza.

39. A) Educate on measures of infection prevention and handwashing.

The patient has a higher risk for infection due to a compromised immune system secondary to corticosteroid use. The nurse should focus on measures that prevent infection, such as handwashing. Educating the patient on the mechanism of action of the medication may be indicated, but it does not help prevent infection and would not be a priority at this time. Antibiotics are primarily used to treat infection, not prevent it. Ambulation is particularly important in postsurgical recovery, but it does not address compromised immunity.

40. A) Obtain a urine sample on the next void.

Symptoms, such as back pain and pain with urination, can indicate a kidney or urinary tract infection; therefore, a urine sample should be obtained for testing. The nurse should encourage the patient to drink fluids and practice good hygiene habits, but this would occur after the proper steps have been taken to obtain a diagnosis. Performing a musculoskeletal examination may be indicated as a secondary intervention; however, the current symptoms are more consistent with a urinary issue.

41. C) "Your kidneys are not producing enough erythropoietin, which helps your body make red blood cells."

The kidneys are responsible for the production of erythropoietin, a hormone that stimulates red blood cell production in the bone marrow. Production of erythropoietin is reduced with chronic kidney disease or kidney failure, so a supplemental form of erythropoietin is usually included in the treatment plan. The kidneys are responsible for maintaining homeostasis but do not regulate the number of circulating red blood cells. The low-phosphorus diet that is recommended for patients on dialysis does not play a direct role in anemia. Although bone marrow dysfunction is involved, the patient's issue is directly related to kidney failure.

42. D) Ask the patient whether he has perianal or rectal pain.

The patient is presenting with signs of an enlarged prostate, which is a typical finding in older male patients and can also occur when a prostate infection is present. Symptoms include difficulty voiding, painful urination, poor urinary stream, abdominal pain, and rectal or perianal pain. Asking whether the patient has perianal or rectal pain can help confirm the suspected prostate issue. Increasing fluid intake will not improve an enlarged prostate and can worsen the abdominal pain if the enlarged prostate is causing bladder distention. Prostate issues cannot be transmitted to others via sexual intercourse, so condom use is not necessary. Performing an abdominal exam is an important step but should be done only after all of the necessary interview questions have been asked.

43. B) Assess vital signs and maintain the safety of the room environment.

An acute change in mental status is not an expected finding after a peritoneal dialysis treatment, and the nurse should evaluate the patient for signs of peritoneal dialysis complications, primarily an infection. Obtaining a full set of vital signs assesses for signs of an infection, so this should be the initial intervention by the nurse. There is no indication that the peritoneal dialysis treatment was not sufficient, so hemodialysis is not warranted. Documenting the findings and performing safety checks do not address the urgent issue the patient is experiencing and would be secondary interventions. The patient is not exhibiting signs of hyperglycemia, so insulin is not indicated at this time.

44. C) "Your call bell should be located next to you at all times, so you can ask for help when you are getting out of bed."
It will be most appropriate for the nurse to discuss the use and location of the call bell, in addition to encouraging the patient to ask for help with position changes and with getting out of bed. Using pillows to block the patient from repositioning during sleep will not prevent falls and may facilitate a fall instead. The nurse should never suggest that the patient urinate in bed unless it is unavoidable because this would contribute to skin breakdown and poor hygiene. Although it is ideal for the patient to maintain the same level of independence as before the hospital admission, this may not always be safe for the patient.

45. A) Schedule repositioning of the patient every 2 hours.
Patients with quadriplegia have impaired mobility and sensory perception; therefore, they cannot feel when ulcerations may be developing. To prevent associated skin breakdown, the most important care plan intervention by the nurse would be to implement repositioning every 2 hours while the patient is in bed or in a chair. Natural sunlight and social interaction in the dining room are both recommended for overall well-being and to help prevent depression, but these interactions are not directly related to the prevention of complications. Although there may be alterations in the patient's temperature perception, the physical temperature of the legs should not differ from that of the rest of the body, so there is no need to check the temperature of the legs.

46. D) Report findings to the medical provider and await new orders.
New onset of visual disturbances in the patient with migraine headaches is an acute change and should be reported immediately to the medical provider. An environment free from bright lights, headache management with acetaminophen, balancing rest with activities, and drinking plenty of fluids are important measures used to treat the migraine, but the immediate need is to assess the new onset of visual disturbances to rule out other possible causes.

47. A) Measuring accurate intake and output values.
Accurate intake and output measurements are important for the newly admitted patient due to the significant loss of fluid that occurs with burns. There are different types of burn dressings, and the timing/frequency of dressing changes will depend on the type of dressing applied. Skin grafts are not initial interventions, and their necessity will be determined by the provider, so there is no need to prepare the patient at this time. Educating the caregiver on the technique of dressing changes would not take place during the initial period.

48. B) Check the current dose and administration schedule for the medication.
To obtain an accurate phenytoin level, the specimen should be drawn based on the time of the last dose of the medication; it should not be automatically drawn at bedtime. Knowing the current medication dose is an important aspect of interpreting the lab result. Fasting is not required for a phenytoin level. The nurse must initially determine the appropriate time to draw the lab specimen; this task cannot be completed immediately.

49. D) Itching in the affected area will resolve after treatment stops, but changes to the skin color may not.

The sites of skin discoloration might be associated with itching during the initial stages of radiation. The itching will resolve, but the skin will not regain its usual color upon completion of therapy. The sites are not usually painful. Although improving daily skin moisture will address skin dryness that contributes to itching sensations, it will have no effect on the appearance of the skin discolorations.

50. B) Reposition the patient in bed, assess the vital signs, and measure amount of gastric output.

The presence of red gastric output is a sign of upper gastrointestinal (GI) bleed and is a medical emergency. The priority actions by the nurse will be to reposition the patient in bed, obtain vital signs to assess for hypovolemia, and measure the amount of gastric output to help determine the amount of bleeding. Once this information is obtained, the nurse should call the provider to discuss the change in status. The gastric tube should not be clamped unless an order is given by the provider. The patient's family should be notified after the immediate care is provided. Intake and output should be assessed as a secondary intervention. Asking the patient to cough and breathe deeply is not appropriate because it does not have any impact on a GI bleed.

51. C) Perform abdominal assessment and report findings to the provider.

Abdominal pain of sudden onset that is excruciating in character is a sign of a medical emergency such as incarcerated hernia, acute appendicitis, or bowel obstruction. To help determine the cause, the nurse should perform an abdominal assessment and report the findings to the medical provider for further instructions. Laxatives should not be administered to a patient with undiagnosed abdominal pain to prevent possible worsening of the condition. Administering pain medications should be postponed until after the abdominal assessment to prevent masking pain, leading to an inaccurate exam. Educating the patient regarding nonpharmacologic techniques should not be performed until the acute issue has been addressed.

52. A) Activate the rapid response team and call the medical provider about the status change.

The patient is exhibiting signs of a stroke, so the nurse will activate the rapid response team and call the medical provider to notify them of the sudden onset of symptoms. Although assessment of gag reflex and accommodation to light may be warranted, this will take place after initiating a rapid response and obtaining orders from the provider. Reviewing the medical records to assess for a cause, obtaining intake and output measurements, and repositioning the patient are all secondary interventions that will take place after the rapid response team is activated and the provider has been notified.

53. B) Use a thickening agent for liquids.
The sores in the mouth cause difficulty in swallowing food and liquid. Therefore, it is recommended to use a thickening agent, which allows better control of liquid in the mouth. Thickening agents help slow down the flow rate of liquids, which lessens the chance of liquid going into the airway. Spicy seasonings should be avoided because they may cause acid reflux, which worsens dysphagia. However, sores in the mouth may result in loss of taste sensation, so non-spicy seasonings are permitted. The sores may cause dry mouth, for which the use of a saliva substitute is highly recommended. The patient should frequently rinse the mouth, which will keep the mouth hydrated and minimize the growth of microorganisms.

54. D) Eat soft, bland, nonacidic foods.
The symptoms of the patient with stomach cancer can be managed by eating soft, bland, and nonacidic food. These types of food prevent pyrosis and ease stomach discomfort. Patients on radiation therapy are instructed to avoid drinking liquid with meals because it makes digestion difficult. These patients are also advised to lie flat after eating for a short duration. Patients having oral cavity problems are typically ordered to avoid commercial mouthwashes; there is no need for such a precaution with stomach cancer.

55. C) "I will avoid taking aspirin for 7 days before the scheduled test."
The patient should avoid any nonsteroidal anti-inflammatory drugs (NSAIDs) for 7 days before the scheduled test; they irritate the gastrointestinal tract, which may interfere with the results of the test by increasing bleeding risk. Aspirin is an NSAID, so the patient's statement regarding avoiding aspirin for 7 days before the scheduled test requires no clarification. It is necessary to avoid vitamin C–rich foods, supplements, and drinks, as well as raw melon, turnips, and radishes, before the scheduled test because they contain peroxidases that can cause false-positive results. The patient must avoid any anticoagulants like warfarin for 7 days before the scheduled test because they can cause false-positive results due to increased bleeding risk.

56. D) Encourage face-to-face conversations with others.
Dysfunction of vocal cords leads to a patient's voice becoming soft or hoarse, which can cause difficulty for others in understanding the person's speech. Therefore, patients diagnosed with vocal cord dysfunction or abnormalities in laryngeal muscles are encouraged to have face-to-face conversations for better understanding. The patient may experience difficulty taking deep breaths while talking in the case of vocal cord dysfunction; however, in cases in which the patient is at risk of hypoxia or its related complications, they are encouraged to take deep breaths because this helps with early detection. The importance of increased rest periods while exercising should be discussed with older patients diagnosed with decreased mobility of the chest wall, but in the case of vocal cord dysfunction, increased rest periods while exercising are not required. Frequent pulmonary hygiene is essential in cases requiring clearance of accumulated mucus. Such cases involve dilation of bronchioles and alveolar ducts, decreased diaphragm strength, and decrease in immunoglobulin A. However, the patient's symptoms are not due to mucus accumulation but to dysfunction of the vocal cords, for which pulmonary hygiene is not required.

57. D) Refrain from smoking for 6 to 8 hours before the test.
A patient who will have a pulmonary function test is asked not to smoke for 6 to 8 hours before the test. Patients should avoid eating before a bronchoscopy, but this is not necessary before a pulmonary function test. The chances of aspiration are high in the case of bronchoscopy due to numbness of the throat, whereas the pulmonary function test is noninvasive with a low risk of aspiration. Because no anesthetics or injected medicines are used during a pulmonary function test, the patient will not experience a stinging sensation. The patient should avoid movement to achieve an accurate result, but deep breathing is required during some portions of the test to determine the functioning of the lungs.

58. C) Frequent coughing.
Pulmonary hygiene involves intentional coughing, postural drainage, percussion, ambulation, and deep breathing. The patient should cough frequently to remove accumulated congestion. The patient should turn and reposition every 1 to 2 hours, not every 3 to 4 hours, to promote patent airway and postural drainage. Lying in the prone position should be recommended because it facilitates postural drainage. Rest is necessary for a quick recovery; however, the patient needs to ambulate and perform activities out of bed, which help in the removal of secretions and facilitate lung expansion. Therefore, the patient should be encouraged to walk without assistance.

59. C) The peristomal area is red and peeling.
A peristomal area that is red and peeling suggests an impairment of skin integrity; this requires a change in the plan of care. The nurse should assess the skin surrounding the stoma and ensure that the pouch system fits properly. Erythema and peeling suggest that the skin is irritated. Cleansing the skin with water, applying a barrier, and creating a properly fitting pouch system can prevent skin breakdown and irritation. A stoma that is pink to dark red and moist indicates that there is adequate circulation to the site. The ileum is the section of the small intestine that is responsible for the absorption of nutrients and vitamins. Water is not absorbed in this region of the intestine; the consistency of the stool should be liquid to pasty. The appliance bag should be deflated before application. If the bag becomes inflated, it is likely due to excess gas accumulation in the bag. The nurse should discuss dietary recommendations with the patient to prevent excess gas.

60. D) "Do you have concerns about changing the bag?"
The nurse needs to validate the patient's feelings and to try to identify barriers or concerns. Understanding why the patient does not want to look at the stoma or change the appliance will allow the nurse to address the patient's concerns and/or perceived barriers. A response of, "I'll do it this time, but you'll have to do it next time," focuses attention on the nurse and does not address the underlying feelings of the patient. In addition, telling the patient that they do not have to change the bag this time promotes avoidance behavior. A response of, "Don't worry, it's simple once you get used to it," does not facilitate communication between the nurse and the patient. The nurse should use therapeutic communication to identify the patient's underlying feelings about managing the ileostomy. It is important to understand why the patient does not want to change the appliance bag and to remove any perceived barriers. "If you change your bag, the doctor will let you go home faster," is not an appropriate response by the nurse because it is a false reassurance statement. Supporting the patient's independence in changing the appliance bag is part of the plan of care; however, other criteria may need to be met for the patient to be discharged.

61. B) "I should clean the skin around the stoma."
The patient should clean the skin around the stoma with lukewarm water to maintain skin integrity. The stoma should be pink and moist and protrude 1 to 3 cm from the abdominal wall. The patient should empty the appliance bag when it is one-third to one-half full. The patient should not insert anything into the stoma; this can irritate and damage the gastrointestinal tract.

62. A) Black coffee
Black coffee is not an appropriate dietary selection for an individual recovering from a duodenal ulcer. The caffeine content in coffee promotes gastric secretions and distress. The nurse should provide additional education to the patient about nutritional intake. A probiotic yogurt shake is an appropriate choice and does not require additional education. Probiotics help restore "good bacteria" in the gut and suppress *Helicobacter pylori*. The patient choosing butternut squash soup would not require additional teaching because the soup is rich in vitamins and fiber, which promote gut health and duodenal ulcer healing. The selection of cranberry juice is appropriate because it contains vitamin C, which promotes healing.

63. C) "I'll let the provider know that you have questions about the procedure."
"I'll let the provider know that you have questions about the procedure" is the appropriate response by the nurse. During the consenting process, the provider should supply information to the patient about the procedure, including medications that may be administered. Endoscopic procedures are generally performed using conscious sedation. Although conscious sedation is intended to block pain, the nurse cannot entirely rule out the possibility of brief pain (e.g., if the initial dosage is insufficient) or other sensation; providing false information can negatively impact the nurse–patient relationship. Specific questions about the procedure should be clarified by the provider. The nurse may not know about medications that will be administered during the procedure, so it is the nurse's responsibility to follow up with the provider and request an additional meeting so the patient's questions can be answered before the procedure occurs.

64. B) White blood cell count 15,000 cells/mm³ (1.5 cells 10⁹/L).
Pantoprazole is a proton pump inhibitor that suppresses gastric secretions. This process increases the patient's susceptibility to infections such as *Clostridium difficile* and pneumonia. An elevated white blood cell count of 15,000 cells/mm³ may indicate an infection. This finding requires follow-up by the nurse. Hemoglobin of 13.0 g/dL, in a patient taking pantoprazole, indicates a therapeutic response to pantoprazole treatment. Female patients experience a normal hemoglobin level between 11 and 15 g/dL. Pantoprazole is a proton pump inhibitor that reduces the production of acid, thereby preventing irritation of the gastrointestinal lining. Proton pump inhibitors can cause elevated blood glucose levels. Therapeutic glucose levels are 70 to 110 mg/dL. Pantoprazole inhibits the gastric secretion production cycle and potentiates the loss of magnesium. This results in decreased serum magnesium levels. The serum magnesium level of 2.0 mEq/L is therapeutic and does not require follow-up by the nurse.

65. A) Administer intravenous loop diuretic.

Patients in Addisonian crisis typically have elevated potassium levels. The nurse should administer an intravenous loop diuretic. Loop diuretics activate the renin–angiotensin–aldosterone system, which blocks transporters from preventing reabsorption of potassium. The nurse should assess heart sounds as part of the assessment, however, the nurse is already aware that the patient is experiencing dysrhythmias, so no nursing action is required. Sodium polystyrene sulfonate binds to potassium and excretes through the stool, but this medication has a delayed onset. The nurse should first administer intravenous furosemide because its onset is 15 to 20 minutes. Monitoring intake and output is part of the treatment plan when managing patients with Addisonian crisis, but this action is not the priority at this time.

66. A) Blood pressure 106/72 mmHg

Individuals experiencing an Addisonian crisis often experience hypotension due to hormone insufficiency. A blood pressure reading of 106/72 mmHg suggests that the patient has adequate perfusion. Addisonian crisis causes decreased aldosterone secretion, resulting in the retention of potassium. Peaked T waves suggest hyperkalemia. The nurse should monitor the patient and implement prescribed interventions to prevent adverse outcomes. Patients with Addisonian crisis experience hypoglycemia because of inadequate hormone production. A blood glucose level of 59 mg/dL (3.3 mmol/L) suggests that the patient is experiencing hypoglycemia and requires intervention by the nurse. Pink and dry mucous membranes suggest dehydration. The nurse should monitor the patient and implement prescribed interventions that support hydration such as oral fluid intake, intravenous fluids, and minimizing fluid loss.

67. B) "At times I should expect to have a fever."

The nurse would need to provide additional education if a patient with Addison's disease is prescribed prednisone and states that at times they will expect to have a fever. Fever may indicate the presence of an infection. Inappropriate management of fever or other illness can result in an Addisonian crisis and rapid deterioration of health status. There is no cure for Addison's disease, and the patient should understand the need to take medication for the rest of their life to manage the disease. Prednisone can increase blood glucose levels. Assessment of blood glucose is recommended to maintain therapeutic levels. Long-term prednisone use can cause bone density loss and early-onset osteoporosis. The provider may monitor the patient with a bone density test.

68. B) Pockets pills in the mouth and coughs after drinking thin liquids.

Pocketing pills in the mouth may be done because of difficulty swallowing pills, and coughing after drinking thin liquids is a possible indication of aspiration. The patient would be placed on nothing-by-mouth status until a speech therapist could perform a swallow evaluation and give recommendations. The patient who swallows pills whole is not exhibiting any signs of swallowing difficulty, and refusing to eat is not necessarily an indication of difficulty. Patients with dementia will often need assistance with eating and setting up their activities; this does not indicate problems with swallowing. Many patients have preferences on how they take their medications and food; these behaviors do not necessarily indicate swallowing problems.

69. B) Reorient the patient to the situation and offer to walk with them.

Kindly reorienting and offering a diversion activity can help patients with dementia to be calmer and more trusting. Telling the patient that they are confused or that they have dementia is demeaning and does not offer a solution, nor does simply telling a patient to stay. Setting the bed alarm is important but does not provide therapeutic communication.

70. B) Ensure that the catheter is patent and unobstructed.

Assessment for physical problems causing the agitation should be addressed first. If a catheter is not draining correctly and urine is backing up in the bladder, this can cause increased agitation. Troubleshooting equipment and addressing all of the things that can be easily and quickly addressed is important in preventing unnecessary interventions. Administering olanzapine or calling a rapid response team would be inappropriate at this time as no other interventions have been implemented. Removal of the catheter is premature; the nurse first needs to establish the reason for the patient's agitation and low output.

71. A) Urine cultures

Results of urine cultures take about 24 hours. Urine cultures are important when treating a UTI in order to treat the patient with the appropriate antibiotics. After obtaining the results, the nurse would notify the provider in case a change in antibiotic is needed. Although monitoring WBC is important, it will not guide the provider in the selection of an antibiotic. *Hemoglobin* refers to the amount of oxygen in red blood cells; it would not be a deciding factor in treatment of an UTI. ALT and AST are liver enzyme values, which do not relate directly to a urinary tract infection.

72. B) Perform a straight catheterization and reassess for continued urinary retention.

Typically, straight catheterization is performed before placing an indwelling catheter. Relieving pressure from a distended bladder often resolves the problem of retention. The nurse would then continue to scan postvoid residuals to monitor for ongoing urinary retention. Indwelling catheterization increases the risk of infection; it should be avoided unless it is needed for strict monitoring, for wound healing, or because straight catheterization has failed to resolve the problem. External suction catheters are used for incontinent patients to help protect their skin. They are an appropriate option for incontinence but would not resolve the problem of retention. Similarly, a brief is used for incontinent patients and would not resolve the retention issue.

73. A) Alert the provider to sudden changes in heart rate.

Ciprofloxacin can cause drug-induced dysrhythmias. Patients taking this drug should be instructed to contact the prescriber if they observe any sudden, unexplained changes in heart rate. Although phenazopyridine causes urine to turn orange in color, color change is not expected with ciprofloxacin. However, dark urine should be reported to the provider because it may indicate liver problems. Antibiotic therapies should be completed for the prescribed amount and time to prevent drug resistance from developing. Administration of ciprofloxacin and antacids should be separated by at least 2 hours to prevent interference of absorption.

74. C) Eliminate sugary foods and drinks.
In addition to prescribed medications, temporary dietary changes to decrease the diarrhea should be implemented until the symptoms resolve. Ingesting any food or drink that has a high sugar content should be avoided because sugar stimulates the gut, which triggers/contributes to diarrhea episodes. A low-fat, low-protein diet would not affect acute, viral diarrhea. Consuming more fiber and roughage will exacerbate the symptoms by increasing gastric motility and frequency of stools. Vitamin supplements do not need to be stopped unless the provider has specifically ordered it for this patient due to secondary reasons.

75. D) Place the patient's arm in a sling.
A flaccid arm must be placed in a sling to protect the extremity and promote proper body mechanics for both the patient and the nurse during transfers. Allowing the arm to dangle freely can place unnecessary strain on the arm and shoulder, resulting in pain and potential damage. Allowing the arm to hang by the side can cause swelling. Strapping an extremity to the core can interfere with mobility. Draping the arm across the body does not provide secure support and impedes proper body mechanics.

76. B) "I should avoid caffeinated beverages."
Caffeinated beverages will contribute to decreased lower esophageal sphincter pressure and will cause increased regurgitation of gastric contents to the esophagus, exacerbating disease symptoms. The acidity of citrus fruits can also exacerbate symptoms. Coughing results from the backflow of acid into the esophagus and is relieved through treatment of the disease and through lifestyle changes, not by taking nebulized medications. Chocolate's acidity can increase symptoms, as does its tendency to lower esophageal sphincter pressure.

77. A) Inspect the stoma daily for discharge and skin integrity.
The patient should inspect the stoma daily for color, type of stool discharge, and intactness of surrounding skin daily. The pouching system may be left in place for showering or bathing. Stoma care should be performed daily and not only when the site is visibly soiled. Positioning in bed will not interfere with stoma patency.

78. A) Stop eating and drinking after midnight the night before the procedure.
The patient should avoid eating and drinking all foods and liquids for several hours before the procedure to minimize the amount of stool in the colon during the procedure. There is no need to avoid solid food for an entire day leading up to the procedure. Because fluids should also be stopped, increasing intake just ahead of the procedure would be inappropriate. Medications, such as laxatives and stool softeners, are prescribed to clear stool from the colon before the procedure, but these medications would be taken 1 to 2 days before the procedure.

79. A) Do not share personal items, utensils, or tableware.
The patient with a diagnosis of viral hepatitis should avoid sharing personal items, utensils, or tableware. Handwashing as a single measure will not effectively prevent spread of disease. The patient who is diagnosed with hepatitis should never donate blood, body organs, or other body tissue. Cooking food with gloves will not prevent spread of the disease as a single measure.

80. A) "Even though my cough is persistent, lack of blood in the sputum means that I do not have cancer."
The development of persistent cough with or without blood in sputum is a warning sign of cancer. Presence of blood-streaked sputum or blood found in a tissue when coughing, and changes in respiratory pattern, are potential signs of lung cancer. The new onset of wheezing and chest pain is a warning sign of lung cancer as well as a sign of acute pulmonary disease requiring medical evaluation; therefore, the patient would be educated to contact the provider right away.

81. C) "The whistling sound is an indicator of breathing too rapidly."
Some inhaler spacers include a whistle. If the patient hears the whistle during administration, the patient is inhaling the medication too quickly. The patient should wait 1 minute between puffs and inhale the medication while firmly pressing down on the canister of the inhaler. The spacer should be cleaned after each use and not only when visibly soiled or dirty.

82. A) Regular exercise will provide health benefits
A regular exercise regimen will assist in maintaining and even enhancing skeletal muscle strength as well as promoting ventilation and perfusion needed for asthma attack prevention. Supplemental oxygen use at bedtime or inhaler use every morning will not prevent asthma attacks. Although outdoor activities can expose patients to triggers for asthma attacks, avoiding outdoor activities completely may not be necessary with proper care and precautions. Additionally, absence of environmental triggers may not be enough to prevent attacks; asthma exacerbation can occur during exposure to stress or increased anxiety.

83. A) "Avoid eating, drinking, and consuming caffeine after midnight."
The nurse will instruct the patient to avoid eating, drinking, or consuming caffeine for several hours before the procedure. Drinking fluids could cause bladder distention, which can cause exacerbation of the condition during the procedure. Having the patient bathe the night before has no impact on the procedure. Reporting any retained metal is a necessary safety precaution prior to MRI procedures.

84. A) Keep all tubing free of kinks to prevent occlusions.
Chest-tube care involves keeping all tubing free of kinks to prevent occlusions, which can prevent adequate drainage. The collection unit should be positioned below the level of the chest tube. Although collection units that use a water seal may exhibit periodic, gentle bubbling, continuous or vigorous bubbling likely indicates an air leak, which must be located and eliminated. When the patient is repositioning in bed, the collection unit should be placed on the side toward which the patient will be turned to prevent accidental dislodgement.

85. C) Right-sided heart failure is characterized by neck vein distention.
Right-sided heart failure is characterized by weight gain, edema, and distended neck veins. Left-sided heart failure is characterized by weak peripheral pulses, oliguria during the day, nocturia, weakness, dizziness, and respiratory distress symptoms.

86. C) Excessive bruising.

Leukemia is characterized by hematuria, ecchymoses, orthostatic hypotension, tachycardia, dyspnea on exertion, and weight loss with anorexia. The patient should be instructed to report any of these to the provider. Increased daytime somnolence and increased thirst are not the characteristics of leukemia.

87. B) Increased creatinine level

Acute-phase rejection occurs in the first 6 months after transplant, and most patients are asymptomatic. If symptoms are present, worsening proteinuria and/or an increase in creatinine level are the most indicative of the acute phase of rejection because they both represent dysfunction within the kidney. A drop in hemoglobin would raise concern for possible bleeding, but it is not directly related to rejection. An erythrocyte sedimentation rate (ESR) can be present whenever inflammation or infection is present; invasive procedures can also cause an increase in ESR without rejection being present. Because there are many reasons why the ESR could be elevated in the patient, this result would not provide a direct link to the acute phase of rejection. Protein, not glucose, as a urinalysis finding would be the most consistent with the acute phase of rejection.

88. B) Check their blood sugar any time they notice that they do not feel well.

Part of patient education includes teaching the patient the symptoms of hypoglycemia and hyperglycemia. In addition to the prescribed schedule for blood glucose checks, the patient should be advised to check their blood glucose level anytime they do not feel well. "Not feeling well" could represent hyperglycemia, hypoglycemia, or an acute illness, which could alter the blood glucose level. Fluctuations in blood sugar levels are expected, and it is impossible for all fluctuations to align with regularly scheduled glucose checks. When sliding-scale insulin is used, the glucose level is checked at the appropriate time and followed immediately by insulin administration that is based on the current result. Administering sliding-scale insulin based on a previous glucose level would cause inaccurate dosing. Meals should be timed in accordance with the patient's lifestyle and prescribed medications such as insulin. If the patient typically eats meals late in the evening and administers their insulin at that time, it would be appropriate to continue late evening meals. Appropriate bedtime snacks are recommended to prevent hypoglycemia at night. Some forms of insulin should be refrigerated, and carrying those insulins on the person would prevent refrigeration. Unnecessarily carrying all insulins also increases the risk for damage to or loss of the medication.

89. A) Perform frequent handwashing.

Cushing's disease weakens the immune system, so frequent and thorough handwashing is required to reduce the risk for infection. Although patients should avoid high-intensity exercise or activities that add significant stress to the skeletal system, they should be taught to engage in regular physical activity of moderate intensity. Patients should follow a normal diet made up of nutritious foods; protein restriction is not necessary. There is no need to avoid outdoor activities provided that they are not high in intensity.

90. D) Obtain weight daily and report more than 2-lb weight gain to the provider.
The patient should obtain daily weight measurements and report increased weight gain of more than 2 lb to the provider. Limitation of free water is not indicated in SIADH, but drinking an increased amount of fluids will exacerbate the course of the disease due to pre-existing hyponatremia. Participation in contact sports and labor-intensive activities will not affect the course of the disease.

91. A) "The balloon at the catheter tip stops the catheter from becoming dislodged."
The balloon at the catheter tip prevents catheter dislodgement. Pulling on the catheter gently is not a way to assess its location. Fluid intake or letting the air out of the urine container will not affect catheter function.

92. A) Sudden, severe pain that is not controlled with pain medications
The nurse should assess for acute compartment syndrome, which is a limb-threatening complication associated with extremity trauma. The "5 Ps" of compartment syndrome include pain, pallor, paresthesia, pulselessness, and paralysis. A sudden onset of severe pain that is not controlled with prescribed pain medications is a sign of compartment syndrome. Given the nature of the injury, any movement, including abduction and adduction, would be expected to result in pain to the extremity. Treatment of the initial injury should involve interventions to minimize swelling, but swelling associated with acute trauma would not rapidly resolve with elevation of the leg. Bruising associated with trauma is an expected finding. The nurse would monitor for rapid worsening of bruising, which would indicate bleeding.

93. A) Perform pelvic floor muscle exercises every day.
The patient should perform pelvic floor muscle exercises daily to strengthen the muscles and improve bladder control. Incontinence pads should be changed frequently to ensure adequate hygiene and prevent skin breakdown due to prolonged exposure to moisture. Although there is no specific number of changes prescribed, one to two changes daily is likely inadequate. Drinking carbonated beverages will not facilitate urination. Self-catheterization should be performed when incomplete bladder emptying is suspected or urine leakage is noted.

94. A) It develops over hours to days.
Delirium develops rapidly over hours to days, unlike conditions such as dementia or depression. There are multiple causes of delirium, though it is most often the result of the patient's underlying condition interacting with a precipitating event. Thinking is disorganized and distorted in delirium; intact thinking with apathy and fatigue is characteristic of depression. A duration of several years is associated with dementia; delirium has a duration of hours to weeks and may resolve when the underlying condition is corrected.

95. A) Abdominal pain
Anticholinesterase drugs, such as neostigmine, are used in the treatment of myasthenia gravis. A risk associated with anticholinesterase drugs is cholinergic crisis; this is often seen when the patient is overmedicated. A cholinergic crisis is characterized by sweating, excessive salivation, bradycardia, nausea, vomiting, abdominal pain, and constricted pupils. The nurse must be able to distinguish these features from a myasthenic crisis, which presents with respiratory distress, increased blood pressure and pulse, and dilated pupils.

96. A) Assess respiratory status.

Tetanus is a medical emergency, and patients are at a high risk for laryngospasm. The nurse should prioritize ensuring satisfactory respiratory function, including a patent airway and adequate breathing. Antibiotics are administered to inhibit further growth of *Clostridium tetani*, the anaerobic bacillus responsible for tetanus. The patient is at risk for seizures, and the nurse can implement precautions after ensuring adequate respiratory function. Any wound should be debrided and any abscess drained, but these tasks can be completed secondary to assessing respiratory status.

97. A) Nasogastric

A nasogastric tube is placed for gastric decompression or short-term feeding due to its large bores and ability to be quickly placed and removed. Nasoduodenal tubes are commonly small bore, which would not be large enough for the removal of the stomach contents during decompression. Gastrostomy tubes and jejunostomy tubes can also be used for feeding and decompression; however, they are surgically placed and are intended for long-term use.

98. C) Recent history of vomiting

Mallory–Weiss tears are most often associated with a recent history of forceful vomiting or coughing; the risk for a Mallory–Weiss tear is increased with long-term alcohol use. Currant jelly–appearing stool is indicative of bleeding at a lower GI source. The nurse would anticipate a normocytic and normochromic anemia related to loss of blood through the GI tract; microcytic anemia is associated with iron-deficiency anemia. The nurse would anticipate decreased urine output and will monitor for signs of shock related to fluid imbalance.

99. A) Sucralfate (Carafate)

Sucralfate (Carafate) acts to form a protective layer and serves as a barrier against acid, bile salts, and enzymes in the stomach. Metoclopramide (Reglan) blocks the effect of dopamine, increases gastric motility and emptying, and reduces reflux. Maalox neutralizes hydrochloric acid but does not form a protective barrier. Lansoprazole (Prevacid) is a proton pump inhibitor that decreases hydrochloric acid secretion, which also decreases irritation of the mucosa but does not form a protective layer.

100. A) Place two large-bore intravenous lines.

The nurse should prioritize airway, breathing, and circulation. Placing two large-bore intravenous lines allows the nurse to start fluid replacement therapy or provide blood transfusions to improve the patient's circulatory status. Monitoring urine output is beneficial for the nurse to assess fluid volume status, but this task can be a secondary priority. A nasogastric tube may be ordered by the provider for treatments such as decompression or lavage, but this is not the nurse's first priority. Specimens for laboratory testing should be obtained after all interventions related to airway, breathing, and circulation have been completed.

101. B) Wait at least 30 seconds after each suctioning pass.
The nurse should wait for at least 30 seconds after each suctioning pass and always hyper-oxygenate for at least 30 seconds between each suctioning pass. The catheter should never be inserted into the tracheostomy with suction already on; suction should be applied intermittently upon withdrawal of the catheter. The nurse should not insert the catheter until meeting resistance (i.e., touching the carina); repeated trauma with the suction catheter can result in damage to the tissue and bleeding. Suctioning the patient's tracheostomy should be completed under sterile technique, not clean technique.

102. C) Check the patient's temperature every 15 to 30 minutes for 1 to 2 hours post procedure.
A sudden temperature spike is a sign of perforation, so the nurse will closely monitor the patient's temperature post procedure. The nurse will prepare the patient for light to moderate sedation and explain that local anesthesia may be sprayed on the throat before insertion of the scope. The nurse will keep the patient nothing by mouth (NPO) for 8 hours before the procedure. After the procedure, the nurse will keep the patient NPO until the gag reflex returns and will monitor bowel sounds per regular protocol.

103. D) Allow only fit-tested employees to care for the patient.
Staff caring for a patient with tuberculosis should wear respirators that have been fit-tested to ensure they mold tightly around the nose and mouth, creating an effective seal. Fit testing should occur yearly or with any significant facial changes, and employees who have not been fit-tested for their mask should not be admitted to the room. A tuberculosis patient should always be placed in a negative-pressure room, which removes contaminated air through exhaust systems and prevents it from flowing outside the room to other patient care areas. Transport should be avoided, if possible, but if necessary the patient may be transported wearing a standard isolation mask to keep from exposing others while outside the negative-pressure room. A Mantoux test is a skin test for diagnosing latent tuberculosis; instead, this patient will likely have a medical workup ordered, including chest x-ray, sputum smear and culture, and appropriate drug therapy.

104. D) Place the wall suction regulator on continuous suction.
The nurse should attach the suction tubing to the regulator via the proper connectors and ensure the chest drainage unit is set at the ordered level of suction. The nurse should never attempt to empty the unit; if it becomes full, the nurse should follow procedure to attach a new unit. The nurse should ensure the patient is receiving continuous suction, not intermittent, and dress or redress the insertion site with an occlusive dressing. Constant bubbling in the water-seal chamber indicates an air leak and requires the nurse to assess for a cause.

105. C) Promote deep breathing and coughing.
The nurse should encourage deep breathing and coughing so the patient has adequate ventilation and is able to clear secretions, decreasing the risk for atelectasis and development of pneumonia. Thoracic binders or strapping the chest with tape should be avoided because these measures limit chest expansion and promote atelectasis. Unless contraindicated, the patient should be placed in a position, such as semi-Fowler's, for easier lung expansion and gas exchange. The patient will need adequate pain management, including nonsteroidal anti-inflammatory drugs (NSAIDs), opioids, or thoracic nerve blocks to minimize pain and allow for adequate deep breathing and coughing.

106. A) Call for help.
A dislodged tracheostomy tube is a medical emergency. The nurse should immediately call for help, stay with the patient, and continue to assess and provide nursing interventions as necessary. The provider or another qualified team member is needed as soon as possible to ensure a patent airway. The nurse should assess the patient's level of consciousness, ability to breathe, and oxygen saturation and the presence of any respiratory distress. A safety kit for emergency reinsertion should always be kept at the bedside; its presence should be periodically confirmed during routine checks so retrieval during an emergency is unnecessary. The nurse should monitor the patient's respiratory status and provide supplemental oxygen as necessary, but only after first calling for help.

107. D) Monitor the patient's temperature.
The nurse should monitor the patient's temperature and the insertion site and assess pain. Arm and shoulder activity on the operative side should be limited to prevent dislodging the leads. The patient is able to be out of bed once stable and is usually discharged the next day; extended bed rest is unnecessary. Adjusting the output or sensitivity is a nursing intervention for patients with temporary pacemakers, not permanent pacemakers.

108. A) Assess cardiopulmonary status.
The nurse should continuously monitor the patient's cardiopulmonary status. The nurse will establish a baseline assessment as the first intervention, so any changes in the patient's condition will be apparent. After that assessment is complete, the nurse will establish and maintain a patent intravenous line for medication and fluid therapy. The patient is at increased risk for injury from a fall related to anticoagulation therapy; appropriate fall precautions should be implemented. The nurse should promote time in a semi-Fowler's position to facilitate breathing, but this would not be the priority nursing intervention.

109. B) Promote early ambulation of the patient.
Early ambulation after VTE results in a more rapid decrease in edema and limb pain. The nurse should never massage over a known VTE site; doing so increases the risk for dislodgement. Warfarin therapy is evaluated by prothrombin time (PT) and international normalized ratio (INR); PTT is used to evaluate and adjust heparin. Leafy, green vegetables are high in vitamin K, which lessens the effect of warfarin. Although moderate consumption of foods containing vitamin K is appropriate, the nurse should not promote increased intake of the vitamin.

110. A) Check the patient's vital signs.
The nurse should assess the patient before performing any other interventions. The nurse will notify the provider as soon as possible after assessing the patient and providing any emergent treatments needed. It is reasonable to reassure the patient that they are being evaluated and cared for; the discharge of a shock feels like a blow to the chest and may cause fear or anxiety. However, it would be inappropriate to tell the patient that nothing is wrong. Obtaining an EKG is a reasonable intervention after ensuring the patient is stable; continuous telemetry is indicated if not initiated before the event.

111. B) Use the mean arterial pressure (MAP) to guide and evaluate treatment.
When treating hypertensive emergencies, the MAP is often used over blood pressure readings alone to guide and evaluate therapy. The blood pressure should be lowered gradually to prevent stroke, myocardial infarction, or renal failure. The patient should remain on bed rest until stabilized to prevent any further increase of blood pressure related to activity. The patient will be transitioned to oral antihypertensives after stabilization of blood pressure with more rapid-acting intravenous medications.

112. A) Place the patient on supplemental oxygen.
Interventions should be prioritized as airway, breathing (oxygenation), and circulation, and then other tasks. Patients with acute coronary syndrome have heart muscle that is becoming hypoxic; the priority intervention is to administer oxygen. Nitroglycerin administration is an intervention that promotes circulation. It is administered to ease angina by increasing vasodilation of the cardiac arteries. Aspirin is given for its antiplatelet mechanism of action to promote perfusion. Morphine may be ordered to reduce pain; breathing may improve when the pain eases, but this would be a secondary effect. Administering oxygen is the primary, direct intervention to improve the patient's breathing.

113. C) Systemic symptoms, such as fever, cough, and nausea, develop.
Stevens–Johnson syndrome is a potentially life-threatening adverse effect of allopurinol. Systemic symptoms, including fever, cough, headache, anorexia, myalgia, and nausea, precede skin and mucosal findings by 1 to 3 days. Symptoms typically occur 4 to 21 days after starting use of the drug. The lesions are extremely painful and usually begin on the palms, soles, and trunk then spread to the face and extremities. Vesicles distributed linearly along a dermatome are consistent with shingles, not Stevens–Johnson syndrome.

114. B) Monitor for behavior changes as a manifestation of pain.
The patient may have difficulty communicating and expressing physical problems. Rely on behavior changes as a clue that the patient may be experiencing pain. Use pureed foods, thickened liquids, and nutritional supplements if chewing and swallowing become problematic for the patient. Liquids (thickened, if necessary) should be offered frequently to promote hydration. Healthcare providers and home caregivers should not correct misstatements or faulty memories and should also avoid criticizing or arguing with the patient.

115. A) Nausea and vomiting
Nausea and vomiting are the most common manifestations of gastrointestinal disease. Anorexia is a lack of appetite and may accompany nausea as a secondary symptom. Heartburn is caused by acid reflux, but this is not the most common manifestation of gastrointestinal disease. Diarrhea is the passage of at least three loose or liquid stools per day and is another symptom of gastrointestinal disease, but it is not the most common.

116. A) Divide meals into six small feedings.

Dumping syndrome is often seen after a gastrectomy. Prevention and treatment of the associated symptoms focus on avoiding triggers that worsen rapid gastric emptying. Meals should be divided into several small feedings to avoid overloading the stomach and intestines, which can result in rapid emptying and associated symptoms such as cramping. Fluids should be given 30 to 45 minutes before or after meals to avoid distention or a feeling of fullness; additional fluids would worsen the symptoms. Avoid offering concentrated sweets, which can give a sense of fullness and trigger gastrointestinal activity. The patient should be encouraged to include soluble fiber in their diet to help slow stomach emptying. Insoluble fiber creates bulk, which can contribute to bloating and cramping.

117. D) *Campylobacter jejuni*

Campylobacter jejuni is a bacterial organism associated with unpasteurized milk and undercooked poultry, making it the most likely cause of the symptoms. *Clostridium difficile* is a contagious bacterial organism that results in severe diarrhea and inflammation of the colon; this bacterial infection most commonly occurs when the normal flora of the colon is altered, such as with antibiotic treatment. *Giardia lamblia* is a highly contagious parasitic organism found in fresh lakes and rivers transmitted via the fecal–oral route. *Entamoeba histolytica* is a parasitic organism transmitted via food, water, or hands contaminated with feces.

118. A) Azotemia

Azotemia, or elevation of blood urea nitrogen (BUN) and serum creatinine levels, is indicative of renal involvement and is a manifestation of acute liver failure (fulminant hepatic failure). Jaundice, a yellowish discoloration of body tissues, is a common manifestation of chronic hepatitis. ALT and AST elevations may be normal in some people, and the elevation of these values is also commonly found in patients with chronic hepatitis. Hepatomegaly, or liver enlargement, is a common manifestation of chronic hepatitis.

119. A) Decreased or absent breath sounds

Atelectasis is a lung condition characterized by collapsed, airless alveoli. Decreased or absent breath sounds are an assessment finding consistent with atelectasis. The nurse would expect the patient to have dullness to percussion over the affected area. Wheezes are consistent with inflammation or narrowing within the airways and are not correlated with atelectasis. The accentuation of the pulmonic heart sound is a manifestation of pulmonary embolism.

120. A) Pneumoconiosis

Pneumoconiosis is a general term for a group of lung diseases caused by inhalation and retention of mineral or metal dust particles. Sarcoidosis is a chronic, multisystem granulomatous disease of unknown origin that primarily affects the lungs. Tuberculosis is an infectious disease caused by *Mycobacterium tuberculosis*. Pleurisy is an inflammation of the pleura caused by infectious diseases, cancer, autoimmune disorders, chest trauma, gastrointestinal disease, and certain medications.

121. A) Auscultate lung sounds

Tension pneumothorax is a medical emergency. The most specific expected assessment finding consistent with tension pneumothorax is decreased or absent breath sounds on the affected side, so the nurse should first assess lung sounds. Hypoxemia, increase in respiratory rate, and diaphoresis are all expected if the patient is experiencing a tension pneumothorax, but these findings are not diagnostic for tension pneumothorax.

122. D) The patient's arterial blood gas shows hypercapnia after 72 hours.

Hypercapnia demonstrated on an arterial blood gas is likely accompanied by acidosis and indicates impaired gas exchange and the retention of carbon dioxide. The patient's respiratory status should be improving by 72 hours. Signs of respiratory acidosis are concerning and require the nurse to intervene. The administration route will be changed to oral when the patient is hemodynamically stable and improving clinically. The patient usually responds to drug therapy within 48 to 72 hours, so 12 hours may be too soon to see improvement and does not indicate the patient is worsening. As the patient improves, the nurse can expect a decrease in temperature, but abnormal physical findings can last more than 7 days.

123. D) Ambulating in the hall with the medical assistant

In addition to antibiotics that treat the underlying condition, a critical component of the treatment of CAP is implementing measures aimed at improving oxygenation. Activities, such as deep breathing, frequent repositioning, incentive spirometer use, and ambulation, all contribute to improved respiratory function because they mobilize lung secretions and prevent further consolidation. With no contraindications present, oral fluid intake should be increased to prevent dehydration and to thin secretions. The supine position places the patient flat, which does not improve oxygenation. The head of bed should be elevated to the patient's comfort. An elevation of 30 to 45 degrees is usually sufficient, but the head of the bed can be raised farther if the patient is experiencing significant respiratory distress. Blood cultures should not be drawn from an existing IV site because pathogens present in the IV and/or the IV tubing will contaminate the test and alter the results of the culture.

124. B) Rifampin

Rifampin may cause an orange discoloration of bodily fluids, such as sputum, urine, sweat, and tears. Although isoniazid, pyrazinamide, and ethambutol may also be used in the treatment of tuberculosis, none will result in the same orange discoloration.

125. A) Dizziness on standing

Orthostatic hypotension should be considered as a possible side effect when planning nursing care. Dry cough is a side effect associated with the administration of angiotensin-converting enzyme (ACE) inhibitors. Bronchospasm is associated with the use of nadolol (Corgard), pindolol (Visken), or propranolol (Inderal), especially in patients with a history of asthma. An expected therapeutic effect of carvedilol (Coreg) is a decreased heart rate. The nurse should monitor for bradycardia as a side effect, not tachycardia.

126. A) Abdominal ascites

When the right ventricle fails, fluid backs up into the venous system, causing the movement of fluid into the tissues and organs. This results in symptoms specific to right-sided heart failure, such as abdominal ascites. Left ventricular hypertrophy is an expected finding consistent with left-sided heart failure. Fluid accumulation in the lungs is a symptom of left-sided heart failure. Poor exercise tolerance and heart dysrhythmias are common in all heart failure patients.

127. C) Absent dorsalis pedis pulses

Absent peripheral pulses should be reported to the provider immediately because this finding is indicative of severely decreased blood flow to the periphery, which can result in tissue necrosis. Proteinuria, or protein in the urine, is an expected finding in a patient with hypertension and does not require an immediate action. Intermittent claudication is muscle pain related to blood flow problems but does not require an immediate action from the nurse. Increased afterload is an expected hemodynamic finding in a patient with hypertension and does not require the nurse's immediate action.

128. A) Hemoglobin (Hgb)

The nurse will monitor Hgb and red blood cell count to evaluate the effectiveness of the iron-replacement therapy because, as anemia is resolving, these levels rise to normal readings. MCV is likely microcytic in iron-deficiency anemia but is not monitored for response to therapy. Serum ferritin levels would not be monitored for response to therapy. TIBC measures the blood's ability to attach itself to iron and transport it around the body and is likely high in iron-deficiency anemia. However, monitoring TIBC is not the best way to assess for response to therapy.

129. A) Iron-deficiency anemia

Iron-deficiency anemia is classified as microcytic (small red blood cell size) and hypochromic (pale color). Vitamin B12 deficiency is characterized by red blood cells that appear macrocytic (large size) and normochromic (normal color). Aplastic anemia and sickle cell anemia both exhibit blood cells that appear normocytic (normal size) and normochromic (normal color).

130. B) Persistent low-grade fever

Due to the pathology of the illness, patients with SCD are considered immunocompromised, so any signs or symptoms of an infectious process should be quickly recognized and addressed. It is important that the nurse understands that SCD patients may not present with typical infectious symptoms; fatigue, malaise, low-grade fever, and loss of appetite are common generic symptoms that may be present with an infection. Anemia is expected with SCD, although sudden, acute worsening of the anemia would be concerning. Patients with SCD experience intermittent pain in the joints; acute onset of severe pain would warrant further investigation. Signs of renal complications of SCD include elevated creatinine; a normal creatinine level is a reassuring finding. If the patient's normal creatinine level became elevated acutely, the nurse should recognize this as an abnormal finding that should be reported to the provider.

131. B) Inspect

The first step to be performed in an abdominal assessment is inspection followed by auscultation, percussion, and then palpation.

132. D) Identify delayed gastric emptying.
Measuring the gastric residual before the next feeding can help to identify gastric emptying. Testing the pH can confirm NG tube placement. Gastric fluid will not be removed for possible irritation. Electrolyte balance is determined by blood testing.

133. C) "My partner will tilt their head forward when swallowing."
During feeding, the patient will keep their head flexed forward to prevent aspiration. The patient will be in the high-Fowler's position, the food will be placed in the unaffected side of the mouth, and the patient will remain upright for at least 30 minutes after eating.

134. A) Obtain vital signs.
Vital signs, especially blood pressure, can be used as a baseline to determine whether the patient is going into shock. Once vital signs are obtained and the patient is stabilized, then pain medication can be administered if ordered, as well as fecal occult blood testing. An upper gastrointestinal series will be ordered after an evaluation by the nurse.

135. D) One half of a chicken breast
One half of a chicken breast contains approximately 26 g of protein. One cup of milk contains approximately 8 g of protein, 1 whole egg contains approximately 6 g protein, and one half-cup cottage cheese contains approximately 15 g of protein.

136. D) Have the patient wear a mask during transport.
Transport of patients with active TB should be limited; when it is necessary, however, the patient should wear a mask to reduce the risk of transmission. Staff should wear fit-tested respirators or N95 (or higher) masks when caring for the patient; a normal surgical mask provides inadequate protection. The patient will be placed in a private, negative-pressure room.

137. C) Actively cough to prevent secretion buildup.
Morphine can cause respiratory depression, which can lead to secretion buildups and blockages. The patient should cough periodically to clear these secretions. Pruritus and constipation are common side effects of morphine and can be treated with medication. Morphine can cause dizziness, and it is important to educate the patient to move slowly while getting out of bed or standing up from a chair.

138. B) Preoxygenate the patient with 100% oxygen.
To prevent hypoxia, the patient needs to be oxygenated before suctioning. Applying suction while advancing can cause trauma to the patient and result in excessive coughing. The suction pass will be limited to 10 to 15 seconds. The nurse will perform no more than three suction passes in order to prevent hypoxia and fatigue.

139. D) Atropine.
Atropine is an anticholinergic used to treat symptomatic bradycardia. Diltiazem is a calcium channel blocker used to treat tachycardia. Metoprolol is a beta-blocker that is used to treat tachycardia. Adenosine is an antiarrhythmic used to treat supraventricular tachycardia.

140. C) Confusion
Signs and symptoms of digoxin toxicity can include confusion, lethargy, diarrhea, nausea and vomiting, vision changes, and poor appetite. The patient would not exhibit increased appetite, constipation, or greater energy.

141. A) Place nonslip socks on the patient's feet.
Wearing nonslip socks will help the patient to maintain temperature comfort and will help prevent falls. Heating pads could cause damage to the skin if the patient cannot feel the temperature properly. The sensation of cold is a localized effect related to inadequate circulation; drinking warm beverages will not resolve the issue. Lanolin can be used to moisturize the dry, flaky skin that can occur with PVD, but it will not help keep the feet warm.

142. A) 4
The transfusion should be completed within 4 hours of the unit's removal from storage. Any longer increases the risk of bacterial growth.

143. D) Be aware that NPH is expected to peak in 4 to 12 hours.
NPH is an intermediate-acting insulin that peaks between 4 and 12 hours. NPH needs to be mixed gently, not vigorously, or it can cause damage to the solution. NPH solution is supposed to be cloudy because it contains a protein called protamine. Unused NPH solution will be stored in the refrigerator, not the freezer, to prevent alteration of the solution.

144. D) Lethargy
When a patient is experiencing anemia from blood loss, they will present with symptoms such as lethargy, hypotension, tachycardia, and decreased appetite.

145. B) Tremors
A patient with hypoglycemia can experience tremors when their blood sugar goes below 70 mg/dL. Increased urination and acetone breath are signs of hyperglycemia, as is tachycardia.

146. D) Check urine for ketones every 4 hours.
Illness increases the risk for DKA in patients with diabetes. The nurse needs to educate the patient on checking the ketones in the urine every 4 hours during illness or when blood glucose is greater than 240 mg/dL. The patient should increase noncaloric fluids, such as water, to maintain blood glucose levels. The patient should check blood glucose levels at least every 4 hours during illness; the provider may recommend more frequent testing. The patient will not stop takin insulin while ill; in fact, they may have to increase it temporarily.

147. B) 9:30 a.m.
Short-acting regular insulin has an onset action of 30 to 60 minutes; therefore, the patient will have a meal in 30 minutes. It takes at least 30 minutes for the insulin to become effective with the absorption of the meal. The patient should not have a meal before 30 minutes have passed or after an hour has passed.

148. B) Place nasal cannula to provide supplemental oxygen.
A patient in sickle cell crisis will need supplemental oxygen because their blood oxygen will be low. This is the priority because this patient is breathing rapidly and experiencing low blood oxygen levels. After supplemental oxygen has been applied, the nurse would start a peripheral IV line to deliver a fluid bolus. This action will address the vital signs and laboratory values showing low blood pressure and poor perfusion to the kidneys. While the fluid bolus is infusing, the nurse would administer pain medication. Asking about the patient's last bowel movement is part of an admission assessment. It is best asked after airway, breathing, and circulation have been addressed and then the patient's pain has been addressed.

149. D) Creatinine of 1.75 mg/dL (154.74 µmol/L)
Creatinine indicates how effectively the kidneys are filtering blood. An elevated creatinine value will appear with AKI. Typically, a creatinine level above 1.5 mg/dL indicates renal injury. Although the other lab values are important, they do not specifically reflect kidney function. Low RBC alone does not indicate AKI. Rather, it indicates anemia, which may be associated with AKI and many other conditions. Elevated WBC does not indicate AKI, but rather infection and inflammation. While elevated WBC may occur in patients experiencing AKI, it also occurs in many other conditions, so it would not lead the nurse to specifically consider AKI. Low hemoglobin levels also indicate anemia, which can be associated with AKI, but this does not explicitly suggest AKI.

150. C) Pale skin and hemoglobin level of 6.5 g/dL (4.03 mmol/L).
Pale skin is an abnormal objective finding related to the low hemoglobin level of 6.5 g/dL. This hemoglobin level indicates that the blood is not being adequately oxygenated. As the patient was admitted with an already low hemoglobin level and is experiencing symptoms, immediate action on a worsening hemoglobin level would be appropriate. The patient's blood pressure (110/64 mmHg) and temperature (98.9°F) are both normal. The respiratory rate (18 breaths/min) is normal, and although the oxygen saturation (93%) is on the lower end, it is much improved from 80% and within defined limits. Urine output above 30 mL/hr and a creatinine value of 1.2 mg/dL are both normal. Although the body may be compensating to keep things within balance, it is important to look at the patient as a whole and to monitor laboratory values for changes. Notifying the doctor of the drop in hemoglobin ensures that interventions can be implemented before something more critical happens.

ANCC Certification Practice Exam

1. The nurse has been assigned four patients. The patient to assess first is the:

   A. 32-year-old postoperative patient, experiencing nausea.
   B. 35-year-old patient post appendectomy, awaiting discharge instructions.
   C. 45-year-old patient with kidney stones, requesting pain medication.
   D. 75-year-old patient with hypertension, reporting chest pain.

2. The nurse is doing rounds after receiving a report on the assigned patient group. The nurse should prioritize seeing the patient:

   A. Whose dressing is saturated with blood.
   B. Whose pulse rate is 90 bpm.
   C. Who has a low-grade fever of 99.9°F (37.7°C).
   D. Who states that they feel nauseated.

3. A patient is reporting postoperative pain, nausea, and vomiting and is experiencing hypotension. The priority nursing diagnosis is:

   A. Acute pain.
   B. Risk for electrolyte imbalance.
   C. Risk for fluid volume deficit.
   D. Risk for infection.

4. The nurse is being assisted by a certified nurse assistant (CNA) while caring for four patients. Which patient need could the nurse delegate to the CNA?

   A. Pain medication
   B. Dressing change
   C. Blood sugar check
   D. Supplemental oxygen for desaturation

5. A patient presents with a potassium level of 2.9 mEq/L (2.9 mmol/L). The continuous intervention that the nurse would ensure is applied includes:

   A. Pulse oximetry.
   B. Bladder irrigation.
   C. Telemetry monitoring.
   D. Video monitoring for safety.

6. The nurse is providing care for a patient post appendectomy. During assessment, the patient reports severe nausea and begins vomiting. Their abdomen is distended and firm, and they deny passing flatus. The conclusion to make after assessment is that:

   A. This is to be expected postoperatively.
   B. The patient is developing an infection.
   C. The patient is developing a postoperative ileus.
   D. The patient is having a reaction to medication.

7. A patient is admitted with a hip fracture, dehydration, and acute kidney injury following a fall in the home. The nurse would expect laboratory values that reflect:

   A. Hyperkalemia.
   B. Hypokalemia.
   C. Hypomagnesemia.
   D. Hyponatremia.

8. A patient has been receiving intravenous fluid replacement for severe dehydration. The nurse is monitoring laboratory values to ensure that the dehydration is improving and is to call the provider for new orders when the serum osmolality is within normal range. The nurse would contact the provider when the patient's osmolarity is:

   A. 200 mOsm/L.
   B. 275 mOsm/L.
   C. 350 mOsm/L.
   D. 425 mOsm/L.

9. The provider has ordered a hypotonic solution for a patient who is severely dehydrated. The nurse would prepare to hang and infuse:

   A. 5% dextrose in Ringer's lactate.
   B. 10% dextrose in water.
   C. 0.9% saline.
   D. 0.45% saline.

10. A patient with hyperparathyroidism has a serum calcium of 12.5 mEq/L (3.12 mmol/L). The nurse would encourage the patient to:

    A. Take a daily calcium supplement.
    B. Drink 3,000 to 4,000 mL/day of fluid.
    C. Take up jogging to strengthen the bones.
    D. Restrict fluid to 1,000 mL/day.

11. A patient admitted for an acute urinary tract infection has a history of congestive heart failure. The provider has ordered normal saline to infuse at 125 mL/hr. After infusion is initiated, the patient reports shortness of breath and has bilateral lower leg +2 edema. The nurse would:

   A. Continue the fluid to resolve the urinary tract infection.
   B. Contact the provider to order a complete blood count to assess for white blood cell count.
   C. Pause the fluids and contact the provider as the patient may be experiencing fluid overload.
   D. Place the patient on continuous telemetry to monitor for arrhythmias.

12. A patient is admitted with diabetic ketoacidosis (DKA). When correcting for hyperglycemia, the provider also orders continuous telemetry. The nurse determines that this order is to monitor for:

   A. Potential ST elevation due to the increased blood sugar.
   B. Atrial fibrillation due to glucose abnormality.
   C. Potential arrhythmias due to hypokalemia when insulin is administered.
   D. Tachycardia due to potential infection from the increased blood sugar.

13. Which cognitive skill of nursing judgment identifies and applies a solution?

   A. Analysis
   B. Assessment
   C. Planning and implementation
   D. Reflecting

14. The nurse hears an intravenous (IV) pump alarming and walks into the room of a patient with thrombophilia to address the alarm. The priority would be to evaluate by:

   A. Assessing the patient and the IV site.
   B. Checking the IV bag to see if it is infusing.
   C. Documenting the IV site.
   D. Silencing the IV pump immediately.

15. The scenario that represents an example of the planning process in nursing care planning is:

   A. Administering an antiemetic to a patient experiencing postoperative vomiting.
   B. Collaborating with the healthcare team to discuss trends of a medically complex patient.
   C. Documenting a sudden change in blood pressure in a patient with dehydration.
   D. Holding a blood pressure medication for a patient experiencing hypotension.

16. Systems thinking includes quality improvement, clinical judgment, patient-centered care, and:

    A. Early warning systems.
    B. Evidence-based practice.
    C. Telehealth.
    D. Therapeutic communication.

17. The nurse is prioritizing patient care. Four patients are in need of attention. Patient 1 needs their Foley catheter emptied. Patient 2 is due for assessment of vital signs. Patient 3 is coughing. Patient 4 is experiencing hypotension with dizziness and nausea. The nurse will prioritize:

    A. Administering cough medicine as needed.
    B. Emptying and recording Foley catheter output.
    C. Obtaining and documenting vital signs.
    D. Administering an intravenous (IV) fluid bolus.

18. The nurse administers intravenous (IV) furosemide (Lasix) to a patient. The outcomes to evaluate whether the medication has been effective are:

    A. Decreased peripheral edema and increased urine output.
    B. Decreased pain and improved appetite.
    C. Decreased urine output and improved mobility.
    D. Increased blood pressure and increased pulse rate.

19. An older adult patient had surgery for a fractured hip due to a fall. The patient is requiring assistance to the restroom and with ambulation. Which patient statement would prompt the nurse to place a referral to care management?

    A. "Getting used to the walker is difficult."
    B. "I feel more painful when I sit too long."
    C. "I'm feeling constipated."
    D. "I live alone; I have no family close by."

20. The pulse rate of a postoperative patient has been increasing over the last 2 hours. Currently, the heart rate is 120 beats/min and sustained. Blood pressure has decreased and is currently 95/55 mmHg with a mean arterial pressure of 68 mmHg. Temperature is 99.5°F (37.5°C), and oxygen saturations are 98% on room air. The urine output in the Foley catheter has had a sudden decrease. Which action would the nurse take first?

    A. Activate the rapid response team.
    B. Call the surgeon and notify of changes.
    C. Continue to monitor for changes.
    D. Place the patient on telemetry monitoring.

21. A patient is receiving intravenous (IV) ketorolac (Toradol) for pain related to an infected wound. Which lab value would alert the nurse to notify the provider for potential alternative treatments to ketorolac?

    A. Creatinine of 1.8 mg/dL (159 μmol/L)
    B. Lactic acid of 1.2 mg/dL (0.13 mmol/L)
    C. Potassium of 4.5 mEq/L (4.5 mmol/L)
    D. White blood cell count of 13,000 cells/m³ (13 cells 10⁹/L)

22. The type of surgical intervention that creates an ileostomy is:

    A. Curative.
    B. Palliative.
    C. Reconstructive.
    D. Transplantation.

23. Following hip surgery, a patient develops sharp pain in their calf. Upon assessment, there is a decrease in pedal pulses, and the leg is hot and tender to the touch. The nurse will:

    A. Ambulate the patient.
    B. Apply cold compression to the leg.
    C. Apply sequential compression devices.
    D. Call provider to place patient on bed rest.

24. A patient is 2 days postoperative. They have been using supplemental oxygen and have now been weaned to room air. During routine vital signs, the patient has a low-grade fever of 99.5°F (37.5°C). The most appropriate first nursing action is to:

    A. Monitor temperature.
    B. Ambulate the patient.
    C. Get the patient a fan.
    D. Encourage incentive spirometer use.

25. The nurse is working the weekend shift taking care of a patient receiving negative pressure dressing therapy. They have a wound vac attached to their wound. The dressings are typically changed on Monday, Wednesday, and Friday. The assessment data indicating that the wound vac dressing needs to be changed today is a(n):

    A. Air leak alarm and loss of suction despite reinforcement.
    B. All black foam covered with transparent tape.
    C. Intact dressing with serosanguinous drainage and continuous suction.
    D. Track pad attached to the black foam.

26. The nurse is assessing the abdominal incision of a postoperative patient. The edges of the incision are separated, and there is no drainage or protrusion from the incision. The nurse would document the wound as:

    A. Approximated.
    B. Clean, dry, intact.
    C. Dehiscence.
    D. Evisceration.

27. The nurse walks into a postoperative patient's room to take vital signs and reassess pain after administering intravenous (IV) morphine. The patient is unresponsive and breathing shallowly at 8 breaths/min. The patient's pulse rate is 100 beats/min, oxygen saturation is 88% on room air, and blood pressure is 115/45 mmHg. The best first action to take is:

    A. Administer naloxone (Narcan).
    B. Apply oxygen.
    C. Call the rapid response team.
    D. Hold the next dose of pain medications.

28. The nurse is providing care for a patient who is post small bowel resection. The symptoms that alert the nurse to potential postoperative ileus are:

    A. Abdominal rigidity, increased pain, hypoactive bowel tones.
    B. Acid reflux, active bowel tones, passing flatus.
    C. Nausea, abdominal tenderness, soft to palpation.
    D. Vomiting, firm distended abdomen, denies flatus.

29. The nurse is providing education on wound care to a patient. To verify that clear information has been provided and to check for any areas that require clarification, the nurse would use:

    A. A written questionnaire.
    B. Closed-ended questions.
    C. The patient interview.
    D. The teach-back method.

30. The nurse recognizes a sign of the patient's low health literacy level when the patient:

    A. Asks a lot of questions of the healthcare team.
    B. Brings their care partner to appointments.
    C. Recognizes pills by appearance rather than label.
    D. Sometimes reschedules appointments.

31. The nurse is providing education on wound care to a patient. To effectively communicate information to the patient during teaching, the nurse should use:

    A. Complex language.
    B. Plain language.
    C. Medical shorthand.
    D. Popular slang.

32. Which phrase requires adjustment based on the need for clear communication in patient teaching?

    A. "Please call your doctor's office for any new bleeding or oozing around the cuts in your belly."
    B. "The percutaneous drain in your abdomen should remain in place for approximately 7 days to prevent postsurgical complications."
    C. "The tube in your belly keeps blood or fluid from collecting where the doctor performed your surgery."
    D. "You should take your new thyroid medicine every morning before you eat or drink anything else."

33. An individual's ability to comprehend basic health information and use it to make decisions that affect their health is known as:

    A. Compliance.
    B. Comprehension.
    C. Cultural competence.
    D. Health literacy.

34. At the completion of patient teaching, what patient response would the nurse interpret as requiring further investigation?

    A. "I will just do what my spouse tells me to do."
    B. "I will take my levothyroxine (Synthroid) as directed on the bottle, one pill each morning on an empty stomach."
    C. "Please give me a second to write that down."
    D. "So, to clarify, I have an appointment this Friday at 10 a.m. with Dr. Smith at his West Boulevard office?"

35. A patient with lupus turns in a health questionnaire partially filled out. The appropriate response from the nurse is:

    A. "Thank you. I'll file this with your chart."
    B. "I'd like to review these questions with you."
    C. "Why didn't you fill this out completely?"
    D. "You must finish this so we can have a thorough history."

36. After teaching a newly diagnosed patient with diabetes about diet modification, the nurse asks, "Do you understand how to choose your foods more appropriately for your blood sugar?" The patient replies, "Yes." To better assess the patient's understanding, the nurse should follow up with:

    A. "Do you think your spouse can make adjustments to your meals to help control your blood sugar?"
    B. "Here is a booklet on the diabetic diet. You should read it and follow it to help reduce your blood sugar."
    C. "Good. So you're not going to eat waffles and syrup anymore for breakfast, right?"
    D. "Will you teach me how you will choose your foods to help manage your blood sugar? Let's start with breakfast as an example."

37. As part of discharge teaching for a postoperative patient, the nurse is discussing handling and emptying of surgical drains. What would the nurse include as the most important infection prevention measure?

    A. Closing drains after emptying
    B. Handwashing
    C. Stripping drains before emptying
    D. Using a new measuring cup every time

38. A respiratory intervention that is critical to teach all postoperative patients in order to address atelectasis and reduce the risk of pneumonia is:

    A. Breathing treatments.
    B. Maintaining nothing-by-mouth status.
    C. Turning, coughing, and deep breathing.
    D. Wearing oxygen.

39. When caring for older postoperative patients, it is important for the nurse to educate the patient on changing positions slowly due to their increased risk of:

    A. Delirium.
    B. Electrolyte imbalances.
    C. Pain.
    D. Postural hypotension.

40. The nurse will educate a patient on the importance of smoking cessation after surgery due to the risk of:

    A. Falls.
    B. Impaired wound healing.
    C. Pain.
    D. Postural hypotension.

41. The nurse is planning education for a patient post hernia repair. To promote the return of bowel function, the nurse would emphasize the importance of:

    A. Ambulation.
    B. Drain maintenance.
    C. Maintaining nothing-by-mouth status.
    D. Incentive spirometry.

42. At the end of an appointment with a patient with diabetes, the nurse makes time for patient teaching. Further teaching would be required if the patient states:

    A. "I file my toenails instead of cutting them."
    B. "I keep my heating pad on my feet at night because it is cold in the house."
    C. "I prefer light socks because they don't make my feet sweat as much."
    D. "I tend to eat lower carbs and more protein with breakfast."

43. Prior to discharge, the nurse gives verbal instruction to a patient and caregiver regarding wound care and medication management and then uses the teach-back method to verify their understanding. The patient and caregiver state that they are confident in performing care following discharge. To supply thorough discharge instruction, the nurse would also provide:

    A. A home health referral.
    B. The patient's belongings.
    C. The patient's discharge medications.
    D. Written instructions.

44. For appropriate patients, a nonpharmacologic intervention that the nurse can offer to increase gut motility and reduce the risk of postoperative ileus is:

    A. Aromatherapy.
    B. Chewing gum.
    C. Incentive spirometer.
    D. Meditation.

45. A patient who underwent an open incisional hernia repair has a midline abdominal incision with staples. The patient has diabetes and has a history of smoking half a pack of cigarettes per day. These risk factors make it a priority to provide discharge teaching on how to prevent, monitor for, and address the potential postsurgical complication of:

    A. Ileus.
    B. Low blood sugar.
    C. Pain.
    D. Wound dehiscence.

46. The nurse is caring for a patient who is currently using a pain relief device that delivers low-voltage electrical current to electrodes attached to the skin. This device is known as a/an:

    A. Electroconvulsive therapy generator.
    B. Intrathecal pain pump.
    C. Spinal cord stimulator.
    D. Transcutaneous electrical nerve stimulation unit.

47. A patient who is sundowning has a recent history of violence. To reduce the need for pharmacologic intervention, the nurse can:

    A. Call security for assistance.
    B. Offer to turn on the patient's favorite music.
    C. Place their hands on the patient's shoulders to provide comforting touch.
    D. Use restraints to control the patient.

48. Which statement by the nurse can help the postoperative patient reduce their risk of ileus, atelectasis and pneumonia, and thrombus formation?

    A. "I am going to help you get up and take a walk around the unit."
    B. "Let me know if your pain is starting to escalate so we can address it."
    C. "We will keep these devices on your legs and turned on while you are in bed."
    D. "You should try to do this breathing exercise 10 times/hr while you're awake."

49. The patient who is post lap cholecystectomy reports nagging pain of 5 out of 10 around the laparoscopic sites that is preventing sleep. They have used the hydrocodone/acetaminophen (Norco) prescribed on the medication administration record (MAR) "for pain of 4-7." They do not want to try the hydromorphone (Dilaudid) that is prescribed "for breakthrough pain of 8-10" because they want to reduce their use of opioids. The patient says the pain is "not that bad; it's just irritating that I can't get comfortable enough to sleep." The nurse will:

    A. Try to find a relaxation or meditation video on the hospital's TV system.
    B. Contact the provider and request stronger pain medication.
    C. Try to convince the patient to take the prescribed hydromorphone (Dilaudid).
    D. Give ibuprofen (Advil), which is listed on the MAR as "for fever >100.5°F," as needed.

50. A complementary, nonpharmacologic therapy that can be used in conjunction with medication management to address both pain and nausea is:

    A. Abdominal binders.
    B. Aromatherapy.
    C. Light-box therapy.
    D. Muscle relaxants.

51. An older adult patient underwent paraesophageal hernia repair and has returned from the recovery area reporting pain of 8 out of 10. The provider's orders are for the patient to remain on nothing-by-mouth (NPO) status until their *upper gastrointestinal series* is completed in the morning. The provider's standard order set contains intramuscular (IM) meperidine (Demerol) "for pain score of 8-10" and oral (PO) hydrocodone/acetaminophen (Norco) "for pain score of 4-7." The appropriate intervention by the nurse is:

    A. Call the provider and request an alternative medication for the patient's pain.
    B. Give the IM meperidine (Demerol) as listed on the medication administration record.
    C. Give the PO hydrocodone/acetaminophen (Norco).
    D. Put on music to distract the patient.

52. A patient is undergoing their first bedside wound vac change and voices that they are "very scared and nervous." The nurse has premedicated the patient per provider's orders. An appropriate intervention is to:

    A. Ask the wound care nurse to come back another time when the patient is not scared.
    B. Call the provider for more pain medication.
    C. Offer to assist the patient with breathing exercises during the dressing change.
    D. Tell the patient the dressing change will be quick and other patients do fine with it.

53. Patients using naproxen for chronic pain should monitor for:

    A. Bleeding.
    B. Body aches.
    C. Constipation.
    D. Cough.

54. What drug class is often added when nonsteroidal anti-inflammatory drugs (NSAIDs) are prescribed to minimize the negative effects of gastrointestinal irritation and ulcers?

    A. Calcium channel blockers
    B. H$_2$ receptor agonists
    C. Laxatives
    D. Opioids

55. The nurse is providing medication education to a patient who has been prescribed an opioid pain medication. The nurse will encourage the patient to incorporate ambulation, increased fluids, and dietary modifications to reduce the risk of what common side effect?

    A. Addiction
    B. Allergic reaction
    C. Constipation
    D. Diarrhea

56. The nurse is providing education to a patient who recently started atorvastatin (Lipitor). What statement will the nurse include?

    A. "Avoid drinking grapefruit juice."
    B. "Take this medication whenever you eat a high-fat meal."
    C. "Take this medication on an empty stomach."
    D. "No dietary adjustments are necessary."

57. A patient is taking warfarin (Coumadin) and has had trouble achieving therapeutic international normalized ratio (INR) and stabilization of the drug dosage in the last month. The nurse will investigate:

    A. Any changes in the patient's sleep patterns.
    B. The patient's consumption of orange juice.
    C. The patient's diet.
    D. The patient's physical activity level.

58. While reporting their health history, the patient with diabetes reports feeling emotionally distressed over recent events in their life. The nurse will demonstrate therapeutic communication effectively during the conversation by:

    A. Actively listening.
    B. Continuing to ask health history–related questions to redirect the patient.
    C. Referring the patient to a mental health counselor.
    D. Using humor to lighten the mood.

59. When developing a plan of care for a 10-year-old patient with autism, the nurse knows it is important to include the parents in the process. The nurse will do this by:

    A. Setting goals for the patient and then sharing them with the parents.
    B. Setting goals with the patient and involving the parents once the goals have been set.
    C. Telling the parents that there is a plan in place and they should not worry.
    D. Working with the parents and patient to set specific goals based on their needs.

60. A patient suddenly becomes tearful over their recent lung cancer diagnosis. They express that they are feeling alone and hopeless. The nurse sits with the patient, allowing them time to reflect. The therapeutic communication technique being demonstrated is:

    A. Clarification.
    B. Informing.
    C. Restating.
    D. Silence.

61. A patient with Crohn's disease is insistent upon using herbal remedies recommended to them by a spiritual healer in their community. Which initial action by the nurse demonstrates appropriate care?

    A. Asking the patient to stop going to the spiritual healer
    B. Explaining the risks associated with herbal remedy use and possible drug interactions
    C. Informing the provider about the herbal remedy use
    D. Taking the herbal remedies away from the patient so they stop using them

62. A patient has just been admitted to the medical–surgical unit with acute appendicitis. During examination, the nurse notices that the patient appears to be anxious. While the nurse is obtaining the patient's health history, the patient reports that they "need God to heal this sickness" and "need lots of prayer." The appropriate response from the nurse is to:

    A. Tell the patient not to worry and that they are in good hands at the hospital, then continue with the health history.
    B. Let the patient know there is a bible by their hospital bed nightstand that they can use if needed.
    C. Ask the patient more questions about their spiritual needs and refer them to the chaplain if the patient agrees.
    D. Ignore the patient's comments because they are not related to health.

63. When caring for a patient with liver cancer who is considering palliative care, which question would the nurse ask to encourage therapeutic communication and help assess goals?

    A. "Are you sure you don't want to continue treatment?"
    B. "Can you tell me more about what you are hoping for with this new plan of care?"
    C. "Did the doctor talk to you about your illness?"
    D. "Do you want to stay at home?"

64. Asking about prior or existing military service should be included as part of the health history intake for new patients because veterans are at an increased risk for:

    A. Posttraumatic stress disorder.

    B. Cardiovascular disease.

    C. Hypertension.

    D. Hyperlipidemia.

65. The preventive health measure considered to be secondary prevention is:

    A. Annual mammograms.

    B. Receiving immunizations.

    C. Using dedicated personal care items.

    D. Washing hands for at least 30 seconds.

66. A patient receiving a blood transfusion containing antibodies will acquire which type of immunity?

    A. Artificial active

    B. Artificial passive

    C. Natural active

    D. Natural passive

67. The nurse is teaching a patient about a heart-healthy lifestyle. A nonmodifiable lifestyle factor would be a:

    A. Thirty-year history of smoking.

    B. Congenital heart defect.

    C. High-sodium, high-fat diet.

    D. Sedentary lifestyle.

68. A patient hospitalized for inpatient chemotherapy is being discharged. The nurse completing the discharge process notices that the immunization screening is not complete. Upon screening, the patient states that they would like any vaccines available to them. What will the nurse do before administering any vaccines?

    A. Choose which vaccines are safe to give and proceed with administration.

    B. Ensure it is safe to administer specific vaccines by checking with the provider.

    C. Give the patient all of the vaccines listed on the screening tool.

    D. Tell the patient they cannot have any vaccines because of their cancer diagnosis.

69. The nurse is educating a patient on the importance of yearly screenings for breast cancer due to a significant familial history. The nurse explains that the cancer of concern is associated with a single gene trait with a 50% chance of passing from generation to generation. This type of genetic disorder is:

    A. Autosomal dominant.

    B. Autosomal recessive.

    C. Complex clustering.

    D. Sex-linked recessive.

70. The nurse reading a patient's tuberculosis (TB) skin test notices a slightly raised, red bump at the site of administration. Which statement by the nurse indicates an appropriate response?

   A. "Have you received the bacille Calmette–Guérin (BCG) vaccine in the past?"
   B. "I will notify the health department of your positive PPD (purified protein derivative) test."
   C. "You're positive for tuberculosis."
   D. "This red bump is pretty small, so I think it's fine."

71. The nurse is admitting a patient who fell at their skilled nursing facility. The patient has dementia and cannot provide an accurate history. Upon physical assessment, the nurse notes brittle hair and nails, skin tenting, and muscle atrophy. The patient is currently on nothing-by-mouth (NPO) status until further testing is completed to determine whether surgical intervention is needed. The nurse will:

   A. Call the provider for orders to change the patient's diet.
   B. Call the patient's family and tell them the facility is mistreating the patient.
   C. Complete a nutrition screening tool and contact the registered dietician per facility protocol.
   D. Do nothing because the patient shows normal signs of aging.

72. Upon discharge, a patient receives a new prescription for simvastatin (Zocor). The nurse will provide medication education along with education regarding:

   A. Depression resources.
   B. Diabetes resources.
   C. Exercise regimen.
   D. Low-residue diet.

73. The nurse is completing the admission for a patient with a history of high cholesterol, high blood pressure, thyroid disorder, and diabetes. The patient states that they take their medications as prescribed and have regular visits with their primary care provider. The patient reports smoking a pack per week of cigarettes, does not drink alcohol, and smokes marijuana a few times a year. They have a supportive spouse with whom they live, and they work full time as a machine operator. The nurse identifies the priority education topic for this patient as:

   A. Calcium-rich diet.
   B. High-fiber diet.
   C. Smoking cessation.
   D. Stress-reduction strategies.

74. A patient has been admitted with symptomatic hemoglobin of 6.9 g/dL (4.28 mmol/L), and the provider orders a blood infusion. At the beginning of the procedure and during the first 15 minutes, it is important for the nurse to:

   A. Assess for changes in energy level.
   B. Draw a repeat hemoglobin blood level.
   C. Monitor and document vital signs.
   D. Measure urine output.

75. The nurse is caring for a patient with frequent, watery stools, abdominal pain, and bloating. The provider has ordered a stool culture and a sensitivity test to rule out *Clostridium difficile* (*C. diff*) infection. The patient's use of which type of medication increases their risk of *C. diff* infection?

    A. Antibiotics
    B. Antiemetics
    C. Beta-blockers
    D. Diuretics

76. Assessment of older adults' nutrition, hydration, mobility, and medication usage is critical for understanding their risk for:

    A. Osteoarthritis.
    B. Constipation.
    C. Decreased sense of taste.
    D. Hearing loss.

77. A pharmaceutical company representative offers to buy all of the nurses lunch in exchange for their providing information about a new diabetes medication to their patients. This is an example of:

    A. Conflict of interest.
    B. Evidence-based practice.
    C. Incentive for working on the unit.
    D. Interprofessional collaboration.

78. The nurse is caring for a patient who is postoperative day 1 from a total thyroidectomy. The patient reports numbness and tingling in their fingertips and around their mouth during breakfast. Vital signs are as follows: heart rate, 62 beats/min; blood pressure, 118/78 mmHg; respiratory rate, 16 breaths/min; O_2 saturation, 98% on room air; and temperature, 98.9°F (37.2°C) orally. The patient describes their pain as a 1/10, and they have no other concerns. The nurse anticipates administering:

    A. Calcium carbonate (Tums) and calcitriol (Rocaltrol).
    B. Ibuprofen (Advil) and gabapentin (Neurontin).
    C. Lisinopril (Prinivil) and hydrochlorothiazide (Microzide).
    D. Oxycodone acetaminophen (Percocet) and docusate sodium (Colace).

79. An older adult patient with altered mental status has been attempting to get out of bed repeatedly. The first thing the nurse should do before deciding whether restraints are warranted is to:

    A. Assess whether risk of injury by not using restraints is greater than risk of using restraints.
    B. Call the patient's family members to notify them of the intended use of restraints.
    C. Call the provider to obtain an order to apply restraints to the patient.
    D. Determine whether the hospital has the appropriate type of restraints in stock.

80. A patient has been admitted with severe diarrhea. The patient is on a telemetry monitor and is exhibiting frequent premature ventricular contractions (PVCs) but is in normal sinus rhythm. The telemetry disruption can be attributed to a lab value of:

    A. Fasting plasma glucose 75 mg/dL (4.16 mmol/L).
    B. Hemoglobin 11.7 g/dL (7.26 mmol/L).
    C. Magnesium 1.2 mg/dL (0.49 mmol/L).
    D. Sodium 134 mEq/L (134 mmol/L).

81. The nurse assessing a patient with Bell's palsy notes impairment of the:

    A. Accessory nerve, cranial nerve XI.
    B. Facial nerve, cranial nerve VII.
    C. Glossopharyngeal nerve, cranial nerve IX.
    D. Trochlear nerve, cranial nerve IV.

82. A patient has been admitted with a gastrointestinal bleed and a positive hemoccult. The patient's hemoglobin is 8.0 g/dL (4.96 mmol/L). Upon assessment, they state that they are a practicing Jehovah's Witness. Based on the patient's statement, the next question the nurse will ask is:

    A. "When was the last time you urinated?"
    B. "Will you receive blood products if you need a blood transfusion?"
    C. "Would you like the hospital's spiritual advisor to visit with you?"
    D. "You are on a clear liquid diet. What would you like to drink?"

83. During health history collection, a patient reports current use of tramadol (Ultram) for the past 6 months following back surgery. The nurse notes that the patient is at risk for:

    A. Constipation.
    B. Diabetes.
    C. Peripheral vascular disease.
    D. Pneumonia.

84. A patient will undergo a CT scan with and without contrast for a suspected renal mass. The nurse immediately notifies the ordering provider when they discover, during health history collection, that the patient is currently taking which medication?

    A. Levothyroxine (Synthroid)
    B. Metformin (Glucophage)
    C. Polyethylene glycol (MiraLAX)
    D. Prednisolone (Omnipred)

85. During an admission health history, the patient reports a troublesome, dry cough for 1 month. The patient reports a history of high blood pressure and gastroesophageal reflux disease (GERD). The nurse will evaluate the patient's medication list for a recent prescription for a(n):

    A. Angiotensin-converting enzyme (ACE) inhibitor.
    B. Antacid.
    C. Diuretic.
    D. Proton pump inhibitor (PPI).

86. The nurse has initiated the first dose of a vancomycin (Vancocin) infusion for the treatment of methicillin-resistant *Staphylococcus aureus* community-acquired pneumonia. Which assessment finding is concerning?

    A. Allergies to azithromycin (Zithromax) 500 mg
    B. Audible crackles in the right lung base
    C. Erythematous rash covering the face and neck
    D. White blood cell count of 15,000 mm³

87. A patient is prescribed intravenous vancomycin (Vancocin) for the treatment of right lower extremity cellulitis. The nurse's priority action before administering the medication is to:

    A. Assess the serum creatinine level.
    B. Check right lower extremity pulses.
    C. Obtain an occult stool sample.
    D. Review the white blood cell count.

88. The nurse is preparing a patient for a nonemergent cardiac catheterization. The patient has a history of high blood pressure, diabetes mellitus type 2, and hyperlipidemia. The nurse would notify the provider if the medication list included:

    A. Amlodipine (Norvasc) 5 mg by mouth daily.
    B. Atorvastatin (Lipitor) 10 mg by mouth at bedtime.
    C. Metformin (Glucophage) ER 500 mg by mouth at bedtime.
    D. One capsule of supplemental fish oil by mouth daily.

89. The priority nursing diagnosis for a patient with a fractured wrist that is in a cast would be:

    A. Risk for disuse syndrome.
    B. Impaired physical mobility.
    C. Acute pain.
    D. Risk for ineffective peripheral perfusion.

90. A patient with paraplegia frequently refuses repositioning and mobility interventions, stating, "I don't understand why these are necessary." The patient is alert and oriented, frequently incontinent of urine and stool, and unable to ambulate. They have a history of pressure injuries. The priority nursing diagnosis for this patient is:

    A. Acute confusion.
    B. Risk for impaired tissue perfusion.
    C. Toileting self-care deficit.
    D. Impaired bed mobility.

91. For which disorder would the nurse assign the nursing diagnosis of dysfunctional gastrointestinal motility?

    A. Appendicitis
    B. Bowel obstruction
    C. Diarrhea
    D. Gallstones

92. A patient is admitted to the medical–surgical unit with a serum sodium level of 125 mEq/L. During fluid replacement, it is most important for the nurse to assess:

    A. Lung sounds.
    B. Dietary intake of sodium.
    C. Neurological status.
    D. Repeat serum sodium levels.

93. The nurse is providing care for a patient who is receiving steroid treatment for exacerbation of chronic obstructive pulmonary disorder. The nurse observes that the patient's blood sugars have been elevated. The priority nursing diagnosis to add to the patient's plan of care is:

    A. Imbalanced nutrition.
    B. Risk for electrolyte imbalance.
    C. Risk for metabolic imbalance syndrome.
    D. Risk for unstable blood glucose.

94. A patient has been tachycardic with a pulse rate as high as 175 bpm. The nurse receives an order for intravenous (IV) metoprolol (Lopressor) as needed (PRN) for a pulse rate of greater than 160 bpm. The patient also has a scheduled oral dose of metoprolol. The appropriate nursing intervention would be to:

    A. Administer both the PRN dose and the scheduled dose.
    B. Administer the scheduled dose.
    C. Call the provider to clarify the order.
    D. Hold both doses.

95. The nurse administers 0.25 mg of intravenous hydromorphone to a postoperative patient for a pain level of 8/10. When the nurse returns 30 minutes later to reassess, the assessment data that indicates that additional intervention for pain may be required is:

    A. Patient ambulating to bathroom, rates pain 5/10.
    B. Patient calm and conversational, rates pain 4/10.
    C. Patient grimacing and tense, pulse rate 105 bpm, rates pain 6/10.
    D. Patient sleeping, breathing 14 breaths/min.

96. A patient has a Jackson–Pratt drain placed postoperatively for an incisional abscess. The nurse is emptying the drain and assessing the output. Which observation would be cause for concern?

    A. 5 mL of serous drainage
    B. 10 mL of purulent drainage
    C. 15 mL of serosanguinous drainage
    D. 80 mL of sanguineous drainage

97. The nurse is obtaining a health history from a patient with cardiovascular disease who does not speak English. The patient is accompanied by their adult child, who speaks limited English. A second adult child, who is fluent in English, is reportedly on the way. Because the nurse speaks only English, the nurse will:

    A. Ask another floor nurse who speaks the patient's primary language for help.
    B. Ask the adult child who is present to interpret.
    C. Wait for the second adult child to arrive and interpret.
    D. Wait for an interpreter from the facility's language service department.

98. A patient presents to the ED with a crushing sensation in the left arm. The patient is short of breath and diaphoretic and reports having consumed a steak dinner with two beers and having taken sildenafil (Viagra) just before the onset of pain. Which intervention is contraindicated in this situation?

    A. Administration of nitroglycerin (Nitrolingual)
    B. Drawing of labs per facility protocol
    C. Initiation of oxygen therapy
    D. Intravenous (IV) fluid therapy

99. The nurse is having difficulty communicating with a patient who has dementia. An aid the nurse can use to facilitate improved communication based on the patient's needs is a(n):

    A. Braille board.
    B. Sound amplifier.
    C. Interpreter.
    D. Picture board.

100. The nurse is preparing to provide wound care to a patient with altered mental status. When entering the patient's room, the nurse notes that they are accompanied by family members. The nurse will:

    A. Introduce themself to the patient and family in the room.
    B. Introduce themself to the patient and begin care.
    C. Talk to the family because the patient's cognition is altered, and they cannot understand.
    D. Proceed directly with care to avoid interrupting the family.

101. A Spanish-speaking patient with diabetes is accompanied by their 12-year-old child, who is there to interpret during the health history intake. The best action for the nurse to take is to:

    A. Ask a Spanish-speaking coworker to interpret instead.
    B. Continue allowing the child to interpret.
    C. Request medical interpreter services.
    D. Use a mobile translation application to communicate with the patient.

102. A patient with lung cancer requests to have no interruptions at specific times through-out the day for prayer. Which nursing principle does the nurse demonstrate best by complying with this request?

    A. Caring for the patient
    B. Cultural competency
    C. Flexibility
    D. Holistic nursing

103. A patient with dementia has multiple family members who visit and make decisions regarding the plan of care. This has been causing confusion among staff members, and some aspects of care have been missed. To advocate for the patient, the initial action the nurse will take to avoid further confusion that may impact the patient's care is to:

    A. Ask the patient which family member they want as their primary decision maker.
    B. Ask the family to identify one family member to communicate with staff.
    C. Help the family to better understand the plan of care.
    D. Tell the family members they must stop visiting because they are causing confusion.

104. During the physical exam of a postoperative thyroidectomy patient, an assessment the nurse will use to evaluate for hypocalcemia is:

    A. Allen's test.
    B. Chvostek's sign.
    C. Montreal Cognitive Assessment.
    D. Romberg test.

105. The nurse is conducting a health history on a patient scheduled for gallbladder sur-gery the next day. When the nurse asks about alcohol consumption, the patient reports that they have drunk a six-pack of beer every evening for the past month. Based on this information, the nurse's priority is to:

    A. Provide information on Alcoholics Anonymous to the patient.
    B. Contact the surgeon; surgery may need to be postponed until the patient has abstained from alcohol.
    C. Review the need for additional laboratory tests to assess the patient's liver function.
    D. Include malnutrition as a nursing diagnosis when developing the care plan for this patient.

106. The priority assessment for the postoperative thyroidectomy patient is:

    A. Airway.
    B. Drain output.
    C. Laboratory values.
    D. Pain.

107. A celebrity has been admitted to the medical–surgical unit after myocardial infarction. Upon leaving the hospital, the nurse is offered $500 by a reporter for details on the celebrity's health status. The nurse knows that if they decide to provide this information, they will be breaching the patient's:

    A. Advance directives.
    B. Plan of care.
    C. Privacy and confidentiality.
    D. Right to information.

108. A newly admitted patient with chest pain has learned they will need to stay overnight to complete a series of tests to help diagnose their condition. The patient reports to the nurse that they do not want to stay in the hospital and that they will follow up with their primary care provider. The patient has a right to:

    A. Require deletion of hospital records.
    B. Have their primary care provider give treatment at the hospital.
    C. Go home for the night and return to their inpatient room tomorrow.
    D. Refuse medical treatment.

109. A patient who is ventilator dependent and can make medical decisions for themself wishes to withdraw from medical care. Their parents, who do not have durable power of attorney, continuously delay withdrawal of care by trying to make this decision for the patient. There are orders to discontinue tube feedings, but the parents ask the nurse to "give the tube feeding anyway." Under these circumstances, the nurse is at risk for:

    A. Lack of autonomy.
    B. Violating privacy rights.
    C. Dishonesty and lack of integrity.
    D. Moral uncertainty and distress.

110. A patient with diabetes asks the nurse whether they can add the nurse on social media. The response from the nurse that will establish healthy boundaries with the patient is:

    A. "No, I don't use social media."
    B. "I'm sorry, but I don't think that would be appropriate."
    C. "Our hospital policy is against patients adding staff on social media."
    D. "Sure, let me give you my information."

111. The patient has decided to receive end-of-life care for stage V renal failure. The nurse does not agree with this decision but will support the patient. This can best be described as:

    A. Demonstrating respect.
    B. Detaching emotionally from the patient.
    C. Keeping personal opinions private.
    D. Overcoming bias.

112. A young patient is scheduled for removal of a uterine cyst. The healthcare provider explains that one of the fallopian tubes is not functioning correctly due to damage from the cyst and recommends removing the fallopian tube, but the patient refuses. Later, the nurse overhears the provider and the patient's spouse in the hallway discussing removal of the tube during surgery without the patient's knowledge. The best initial action for the nurse to take is to:

    A. Confront the spouse about the discussion.

    B. Do nothing because the provider has more authority.

    C. Have a conversation with the patient about what was witnessed.

    D. Report the incident to the hospital ethics committee.

113. The nurse notes acute changes in a patient's respiratory status, including an increased respiratory rate, shallow respirations, moist crackles on auscultation, and patient report of shortness of breath. The nurse recognizes these symptoms as clinical indications of:

    A. Emphysema.

    B. Fluid overload.

    C. Pleurisy.

    D. Tuberculosis.

114. A patient with emphysema shouts every time the provider walks by the room because they are upset with their plan of care and treatment. Their behavior is making the nurse anxious, and other nurses have reported delaying going into the room because of the patient's behavior. As a result, medications have been administered late, and the patient is not receiving optimal care. The best action the nurse can take is:

    A. Asking the provider to discharge the patient because of their behavior.

    B. Continuing delaying care until the patient has calmed down.

    C. Having a conversation with the patient about their behavior.

    D. Having security accompany them to the room each time they provide care.

115. The nurse will ensure accurate daily weights using the same scale and weighing a patient at the same time each day because weight is the most reliable indicator of:

    A. Blood sugar.

    B. Electrolytes.

    C. Fluid balance.

    D. Infection.

116. A patient with liver failure has ascites. Assessment reveals fluid retention. The type of diet the nurse will implement is:

    A. Low cholesterol.

    B. Low fiber.

    C. Sodium restricted.

    D. Vegetarian.

117. A patient who just completed their first ultra-marathon (100 km race) is admitted with severe muscle pain, dark urine, and low urine output. The nurse recognizes these as indications of:

    A. Gout.
    B. Muscle atrophy.
    C. Rhabdomyolysis.
    D. Urinary tract infection.

118. While changing a patient's ileostomy pouch, the nurse notes redness and excoriation of the skin around the stoma. To prevent further breakdown of the skin around the new ostomy appliance, the nurse will:

    A. Apply a skin barrier and verify correct sizing of the appliance.
    B. Change the new appliance frequently.
    C. Reduce the frequency of emptying the ostomy pouch.
    D. Remove the appliance and cover the stoma with a dressing.

119. The nurse observes a patient having an abrupt loss of muscle tone and function that lasts only a few seconds and is followed by the patient being confused about what occurred. The nurse suspects the patient has experienced a(n):

    A. Atonic seizure.
    B. Aura.
    C. Clonic seizure.
    D. Myoclonic seizure.

120. The nurse's assessment of a patient with a brain injury reveals abnormal posturing of the body. The arms and hands are noted to be bent in toward the body, while the legs are straightened with the toes pointed downward. This posture is known as:

    A. Clonus.
    B. Decerebrate posture.
    C. Decorticate posture.
    D. Tripod position.

121. A patient with diabetes has been dependent on insulin for more than 30 years. The laboratory value that indicates that the patient is maintaining overall euglycemia with their current insulin regimen is:

    A. Blood urea nitrogen (BUN) 18 mg/dL (6.43 mmol/L).
    B. Calcium 8.6 mg/dL (2.15 mmol/L).
    C. Fasting plasma glucose 134 mg/dL (7.44 mmol/L).
    D. Glycated hemoglobin (glycohemoglobin A1C) 5.3% (53 g/L).

122. A patient is admitted to the medical–surgical unit with complications from metastatic colon cancer chemotherapy. The patient has had several courses of radiation and chemotherapy over the past several years. They disclose that they are "tired of needles and would like to go peacefully." The nurse will:

    A. Administer pain medication to the patient as needed.
    B. Ask the patient whether they would like a family meeting with the provider to discuss goals of care.
    C. Ask the patient whether they would like the lights dimmed so that they can take a restful nap.
    D. Tell the patient that it is important for them to keep a positive attitude.

123. A patient with diabetes has been dependent on insulin for more than 25 years and is being admitted with diabetic ketoacidosis. The nurse's admission assessment reveals that the patient lives alone without support. The patient states upon admission that "everything is blurry." Upon further assessment, they are not able to see the syringe markings and have not been administering accurate insulin doses. The nurse will:

    A. Ask the patient what diet they are following.
    B. Ask the provider whether the patient can switch to an oral diabetic agent.
    C. Consult with case management to arrange home medication assistance on discharge.
    D. Educate the patient on insulin compliance.

124. The nurse is caring for a patient with cardiovascular disease. The nurse wishes to collect subjective data from the patient. The type of questioning the nurse will use is:

    A. Inference.
    B. Laundry list.
    C. Leading questions.
    D. Open-ended questions.

125. A patient's medication list is an important part of the health history. Which medications, if used by a patient preoperatively, may negatively affect the patient's postoperative wound healing and fluid and electrolyte balance?

    A. Corticosteroids
    B. Insulins
    C. Thyroid medications
    D. Vitamins

126. When obtaining a health history from a patient with diabetes, the communication technique the nurse uses when they need clarification of the patient's response is:

    A. Active listening.
    B. Nonverbal communication.
    C. Rephrasing.
    D. Silence.

127. A patient reports a cut on their lower leg that they have been bandaging for 2 months after a fall. The other disease history the nurse will need to thoroughly assess for is:

   A. Alzheimer's disease.
   B. Diabetes mellitus.
   C. Herpes zoster.
   D. Seizures.

128. The nurse is caring for a patient experiencing hyponatremia. Which lab value should the nurse monitor?

   A. Potassium
   B. Calcium
   C. Sodium
   D. Vitamin K

129. The nurse is caring for a patient with lupus who has been admitted for suicidal ideation. A question included in the nurse's initial assessment is:

   A. "Why are you trying to harm yourself?"
   B. "What makes you so upset?"
   C. "Do you have a plan to harm yourself?"
   D. "Why do you think cutting your wrists will make things better?"

130. A patient diagnosed with congestive heart failure has brain natriuretic peptide (BNP) greater than 5,000 ng/L. There are audible crackles in the bilateral lower bases of the lungs and pitting edema in the bilateral lower extremities. The patient's ejection fraction is 40%. The order the nurse anticipates is:

   A. Administer 0.9% normal saline infusion at 100 mL/hr.
   B. Implement a high-sodium diet protocol.
   C. Maintain fluid restriction of 4,000 mL/day.
   D. Push furosemide 40 mg intravenously.

131. The nurse is assessing the patient's likelihood of falling. The tool the nurse will use is the:

   A. Braden scale.
   B. Glasgow scale.
   C. Morse scale.
   D. Wong–Baker FACES scale.

132. The nurse working in the acute care hospital implements fall precautions for a patient with dementia. The nurse will:

   A. Decrease the height of the bed to the lowest position.
   B. Elevate all four side rails of the bed before leaving the patient's room.
   C. Remove personal items from the bedside table.
   D. Unplug the bed alarm after performing patient care.

133. The nurse is caring for a patient prescribed vancomycin (Vancocin). The patient has begun experiencing foul-smelling diarrhea. The priority recommendation the nurse makes to the provider is:

    A. Increase the vancomycin dose.
    B. Obtain a stool sample.
    C. Add administration of intravenous fluids.
    D. Order an antidiarrheal.

134. The nurse is reviewing laboratory results in the electronic health record. Which value is out of range?

    A. Serum calcium 9.2 mg/dL
    B. Serum magnesium 2.0 mEq/L
    C. Serum potassium 5.5 mEq/L
    D. Serum sodium 138 mEq/L

135. The nurse is caring for a patient with lung cancer who is on suicide precautions. The finding that poses a risk to the patient's safety is that:

    A. The patient is placed in a room with nonescape windows.
    B. A healthcare sitter is in the patient's assigned room.
    C. Dietary staff remove plastic utensils from the patient's tray.
    D. A sharps container is located on the wall near the door entry.

136. The nurse notices that the patient's serum creatinine level is elevated. The nurse uses this value to assess function of what organ?

    A. Heart
    B. Kidney
    C. Lung
    D. Spleen

137. The nurse is caring for an older adult diagnosed with dementia and wants to use restraint alternatives. Which selection achieves this goal?

    A. Give the patient a blanket to fold.
    B. Lock the patient in a quiet room alone.
    C. Place mitts on the patient's hands.
    D. Tie the patient with a quick-release knot to the bedframe.

138. A patient admitted for uncontrolled diabetes mellitus appears diaphoretic and exhibits a change in mentation. Point-of-care testing reveals a low blood glucose level. The nurse will:

    A. Administer a basal dose of insulin aspart (NovoLog) 5 units.
    B. Conduct an in-depth neurologic assessment.
    C. Intravenously push an amp of 50% dextrose (D50).
    D. Place a cool, damp towel on the patient's forehead.

139. The nurse is admitting a patient who reports fever, chills, night sweats, and hemoptysis for 3 months. Which action will the nurse perform first?

    A. Administer intravenous antibiotics to the patient.
    B. Apply airborne precaution personal protective equipment.
    C. Have the patient consent to thoracentesis.
    D. Obtain a sputum culture from the patient.

140. The nurse is completing an admission assessment for a patient with pneumonia who has been recently admitted to the medical–surgical unit. The nurse should initiate safety precautions against falls if the assessment reveals that the patient:

    A. Fell at home 1 month ago.
    B. Uses a wheelchair.
    C. Has a history of asthma.
    D. Wants to wear nonskid shoes.

141. The nurse is caring for a patient who is confused and is receiving antibiotic therapy. The nurse has applied restraints to the patient's wrist to prevent central line dislodgement. An additional intervention to add to the patient's plan of care is:

    A. Assess the peripheral pulses.
    B. Place the patient in a supine position.
    C. Request a nothing-by-mouth (NPO) order.
    D. Tie the restraints to the bedrail.

142. The nurse is caring for a patient who has a leg wound colonized with methicillin-resistant *Staphylococcus aureus*. Before performing wound care, the nurse applies gloves and a/an:

    A. Face shield.
    B. Gown.
    C. N95 respirator.
    D. Surgical mask.

143. A patient with a recent myocardial infarction states, "I don't care about attending cardiac rehabilitation classes. My life is over, and nothing will help." The nurse will:

    A. Administer pain medication as needed to ease the patient's feelings.
    B. Tell the patient, "Being negative won't help."
    C. Respond, "Maybe you'll feel better after getting some rest."
    D. Let the provider know the patient may need depression screening.

144. The nurse is caring for a 20-year-old university student who reports sudden onset of neck rigidity and has an oral temperature of 102.4°F (39.1°C). The personal protective equipment the nurse must obtain from the supply closet includes:

    A. Gloves, face shield, and gown.
    B. Gown, gloves, and N95 respirator.
    C. N95 respirator, face shield, and gloves.
    D. Surgical mask, gown, and gloves.

145. A patient has been in the ICU for 10 days and is now transferred to the medical–surgical floor. The patient was previously alert and oriented. The patient now reports seeing insects that are not present in the room and is not able to state where they are. The nurse will:

    A. Encourage the patient to sleep for the rest of the day.
    B. Suspect hospital delirium and incorporate interventions.
    C. Ask the patient's spouse to stay in the room to provide company.
    D. Tell the patient there are no bugs in the room and continue with care.

146. A patient recently diagnosed with Parkinson's disease is receiving education regarding carbidopa and levodopa (Sinemet). They say, "I will take this medication and I will be cured." The nurse will:

    A. Document successful medication education.
    B. Educate the patient that this medication only assists with symptoms.
    C. Ensure that the patient knows to take the medication at least once a week.
    D. Tell the patient they should not be so confident about the medication.

147. A patient with a history of dementia is 1 day postoperative from hip surgery, disoriented, and not able to state needs. To accurately assess pain, the nurse will:

    A. Ask the patient their pain number on the numeric 1 to 10 scale.
    B. Document that the patient is in no pain because the patient does not say they are in pain.
    C. Use the FACES pain rating scale.
    D. Use the Pain Assessment in Advanced Dementia (PAINAD) scale for observational assessment.

148. An older adult patient has been admitted after a fall with no diagnosed head injury, and they have just finished breakfast. After the nurse enters the room, the patient states, "When is breakfast?" The conclusion the nurse would make is that the patient:

    A. Is still hungry and another breakfast is indicated.
    B. Has short-term memory issues and needs frequent reorientation.
    C. Is experiencing a stroke.
    D. Needs their blood glucose assessed because it may be low.

149. The nursing diagnosis to prioritize is:

    A. Risk for decreased circulation.
    B. Risk for inadequate nutrition intake.
    C. Ineffective airway clearance.
    D. Ineffective breathing pattern.

150. During an annual physical, a patient reports a history of frequent job changes and alcohol use. The patient is very fidgety, appears to be having difficulty concentrating, and is easily distracted. The nurse will:

A. Tell the patient to calm down and pay attention.

B. Ask why the patient cannot maintain employment.

C. Perform a complete physical assessment, including heart and lung sounds.

D. Ask whether the patient has ever been assessed for attention deficit disorder (ADD).

ANCC Certification Practice Exam: Answers

1. D) 75-year-old patient with hypertension, reporting chest pain.
The nurse should always address airway, breathing, and circulation problems first, then move through other issues. A patient experiencing chest pain needs immediate evaluation and, potentially, interventions to save cardiac cells. This situation would necessitate rapid response team involvement. Postoperative nausea is common and should be addressed quickly to facilitate the recovery process. Kidney stones accompanied by pain should be addressed quickly. Pain should be addressed within 15 minutes of the patient requesting medication. A patient awaiting discharge instructions is stable and can be addressed last.

2. A) Whose dressing is saturated with blood.
When prioritizing patient care, nurses should work from the most life-threatening to the least life-threatening event. Airway, breathing, and circulation should always be prioritized. Symptoms that are sudden changes or that need intervention should be addressed next. A dressing saturated with blood should be assessed first to see the extent of bleeding. A pulse rate of 90 bpm is within the normal range (i.e., between 60 bpm and 100 bpm). The patient with low-grade fever should be monitored; medications are typically ordered for temperatures greater than 101°F (38.3°C). Nausea should be addressed, but it is a lower priority than bleeding.

3. C) Risk for fluid volume deficit.
Fluid volume deficit occurs when the blood volume drops quickly and the body is unable to compensate. It can be caused by vomiting or dehydration. This patient is experiencing hypotension accompanied by vomiting, which increases fluid loss. When there is inadequate fluid volume (i.e., low blood pressure), there is an increased risk for lack of oxygenation and perfusion as well. Therefore, blood pressure would be a priority to address. Pain should be addressed as promptly as possible, but fluid deficit is a higher priority. Electrolyte imbalance occurs with the deficit or excess of fluid volume and can cause dysrhythmias, but imbalances can be corrected after the deficit is addressed. There is no indication of increased risk for infection.

4. C) Blood sugar check
A nurse can delegate certain tasks. A blood sugar check can be delegated because it is a task that the CNA can perform. The result should be reported back to the nurse. Assessment, interventions, and documentation should never be delegated. Any tasks delegated should be followed up by the nurse. Medications and dressing changes cannot be delegated. A patient who is desaturating needs further assessment from the nurse.

5. C) Telemetry monitoring.

The patient is exhibiting hypokalemia (potassium level below 3.5 mEq/L). Because hypokalemia presents the risk for lethal arrhythmias, the patient requires continuous cardiac monitoring. Pulse oximetry is not necessary because potassium does not interfere with oxygenation. Bladder irrigation does not impact potassium. Video monitoring is usually used if a patient is at a high fall risk and is confused, but it is unnecessary for a patient with low potassium.

6. C) The patient is developing a postoperative ileus.

A postoperative ileus is the lack of motility in the gastrointestinal tract following surgery. The symptoms include nausea, vomiting with oral intake, and a distended and firm abdomen. An ileus is a complication of surgery and should be addressed promptly. An infection would be seen through tachycardia, hypotension, fever, and increased white blood cells count. Medication reactions occur shortly after medication administration.

7. A) Hyperkalemia.

Hyperkalemia is seen in instances of dehydration and kidney injury. In these instances, the fluid volume makes the blood chemistry more concentrated. Hypokalemia is seen in fluid overload and alkalosis. Hypomagnesemia is seen with malnutrition and alcoholism. Hyponatremia is seen in liver disease and adrenal insufficiency.

8. B) 275 mOsm/L.

The nurse would call for new orders when the patient's osmolarity is 275 mOsm/L. Normal serum osmolarity is between 270 and 300 mOsm/L, and anything in that range is considered isotonic. Anything below 270 mOsm/L is considered hypotonic. Results above 300 are considered hypertonic.

9. D) 0.45% saline.

The 0.45% saline is a hypotonic solution, meaning it has less than normal serum osmolality. Five percent dextrose in Ringer's lactate is a hypertonic solution, meaning it is more concentrated than normal serum osmolality. Ten percent dextrose is also a hypertonic solution. The 0.9% saline is an isotonic solution, meaning is has normal serum osmolality.

10. B) Drink 3,000 to 4,000 mL/day of fluid.

The patient is exhibiting hypercalcemia, so the nurse would encourage fluids to flush the excess calcium from the body through the kidneys. The nurse should not encourage calcium supplementation if the calcium level is already high. Ambulation is encouraged, but patients with this disease have an increased risk of pathologic fractures and weakness; jogging presents the risk of injury and falls. Fluids should be encouraged, not restricted.

11. C) Pause the fluids and contact the provider as the patient may be experiencing fluid overload.

The patient is exhibiting signs of fluid overload, which requires intervention. It is prudent to pause the intravenous fluids and call the provider to notify of symptoms. Fluids will not resolve the infection; the patient requires antibiotics. Knowing the white blood cell count would not help address fluid overload. The patient would not need to be placed on telemetry for fluid overload.

12. C) Potential arrhythmias due to hypokalemia when insulin is administered.
When insulin is administered to treat the hyperglycemia, the insulin drives potassium into the cells and may cause hypokalemia. Therefore, the patient will be monitored for potential arrhythmias. The patient would not be at risk for a myocardial infarction or ST elevation. DKA does not cause atrial fibrillation. The patient is at risk for infection with increased blood sugar, but this would not be a reason to place the patient on telemetry.

13. C) Planning and implementation
Planning and implementation refers to creating solutions and implementing them. *Analysis* refers to interpreting data and brainstorming; it is the basis for planning. *Assessment* refers to collecting data. *Reflecting* refers to deciding whether the interventions are working or need revamping.

14. A) Assessing the patient and the IV site.
The nurse would assess the patient and the IV site first. Whenever the nurse enters a room, the patient should be the priority. Assessing the patient and the IV site can signal the nurse to any complications. Checking the IV bag to see whether it is infusing is also appropriate but is not the priority. Documenting the IV site would be done last, after the evaluation has been completed. Silencing the pump is appropriate after the patient has been evaluated.

15. B) Collaborating with the healthcare team to discuss trends of a medically complex patient.
Collaboration is part of the planning process. Meeting with the entire healthcare team, including the provider, social worker, physical therapist, and occupational therapist, regarding trends and data of a medically complex patient allows the team to coordinate and plan the best care. Administering an antiemetic to a patient experiencing postoperative vomiting would be an example of implementation. Documenting a sudden change in blood pressure in a patient with dehydration is an example of evaluation. Holding a blood pressure medication for a patient experiencing hypotension is an example of implementation and evaluation at the same time.

16. B) Evidence-based practice.
Evidence-based practice is part of systems thinking and should be applied to the nurse's clinical practice. Early warning signs are assessment data that forecast changes. Telehealth is healthcare delivered via electronics. Therapeutic communication is a considerate and sensitive style of interacting with patients.

17. D) Administering an intravenous (IV) fluid bolus.
A patient experiencing symptomatic hypotension requires immediate intervention; therefore, administering an IV fluid bolus for Patient 4 would be the priority nursing intervention. Emptying catheters and taking vital signs are tasks that can be delegated to a certified nursing assistant. Administering an as-needed cough medicine is a lower priority than addressing blood pressure.

18. A) Decreased peripheral edema and increased urine output.
The nurse would evaluate the patient for decreased peripheral edema and increased urine output. IV furosemide should pull excess water away from the interstitial space and excrete it through the kidneys as increased urine. There should also be a noticeable decrease in edema. Pain and appetite are not directly affected by furosemide. Urine output should increase, not decrease. Mobility is not directly affected by the use of furosemide. Blood pressure should decrease with use of furosemide, not increase. An increased pulse rate alone would not indicate that IV furosemide has been effective.

19. D) "I live alone; I have no family close by."
This patient needs assistance with activities of daily living, such as ambulation and getting to the bathroom. If they live alone and have no family close by to provide the assistance, collaboration with care management would be an important part of planning for a safe discharge. "Getting used to the walker is difficult" would prompt some additional patient education regarding proper use of the walker and potential collaboration with physical therapy. "I feel more painful when I sit too long" would also prompt some additional patient education as well as suggesting other nursing interventions, such as ice application, elevation of the legs, and frequent position changes. "I'm feeling constipated" would prompt the nurse to implement an intervention such as stool softeners or a suppository.

20. A) Activate the rapid response team.
When a patient's status changes drastically for the worse, it is best to collaborate. Activating and collaborating with a rapid response team can prevent complications from the deteriorating status of the patient and aid in early interventions. The nurse would notify the surgeon, but involving a rapid response team can get interventions rolling quicker. The patient requires immediate interventions to help their deteriorating condition; continuing to monitor the changes would not be appropriate at this time. Placing the patient on telemetry may be required but is only a small piece of the interventions that need to happen.

21. A) Creatinine of 1.8 mg/dL (159 μmol/L)
Elevated creatinine points to acute kidney injury. IV ketorolac can directly affect kidney function. A creatinine level of greater than 1.2 for women and greater than 1.4 for men may be an early sign that the kidneys are not working properly. Lactic acid is a sepsis marker and would not be affected by IV ketorolac. Potassium is an electrolyte; it is affected by some diuretics, but ketorolac is not expected to affect potassium level or increase risk of infection. White blood cell count indicates infection. It is often addressed by antibiotic therapy.

22. B) Palliative.
Palliative surgery refers to a surgical intervention performed to remove chronic discomfort. An ileostomy is the creation of an opening in the abdominal wall for the purpose of emptying fecal matter. Crohn's disease, cancer, and toxic megacolon are some conditions for which an ileostomy would be considered to relieve chronic pain and bowel complications. Curative surgery is a surgical intervention that addresses the cause of illness. *Reconstructive surgery* refers to the repair or replacement of a body part that was not functioning properly. *Transplantation* refers to replacing a body part with a transplant.

23. D) Call provider to place patient on bed rest.

Signs and symptoms of deep vein thrombosis (DVT) include localized pain, edema, redness, heat, and decreased distal pulses. If a DVT is suspected, the provider should be notified and the patient placed on bed rest until a duplex scan has confirmed the DVT. This is because there is a risk of dislodging a DVT and its traveling to the lungs and becoming a pulmonary embolism. Ambulating the patient, applying cold compression, and applying sequential compression devices are not appropriate interventions when a DVT is suspected.

24. D) Encourage incentive spirometer use.

The priority is to teach and encourage the use of incentive spirometry as a proactive step toward preventing postoperative complications. The patient needs to do deep-breathing exercises to increase gas exchange. Shallow or weak breathing can increase body temperature. Encouraging the patient to do some breathing exercise with the use of an incentive spirometer would be the most appropriate first action. The nurse will continue to monitor the patient and can recheck the patient's temperature after the patient completes deep-breathing exercises. Ambulating the patient is important and can help in deeper breathing; however, the incentive spirometer is a more readily available intervention. Getting a fan is also appropriate, but using the incentive spirometer is more appropriate.

25. A) Air leak alarm and loss of suction despite reinforcement.

If the wound vac is alarming and notifying of an air leak, reinforcing it is appropriate. If, after reinforcement of the leak, there continues to be loss of suction, the nurse should replace the wound vac dressing. A well-functioning wound vac dressing should be intact, the track pad attached to the black foam for suction, and all black foam covered with transparent tape. A dressing that loses suction despite being reinforced with additional tape needs to be replaced so that the patient receives the benefit of the negative pressure.

26. C) Dehiscence.

Dehiscence is the term used to describe separated edges of a surgical incision. If the edges of the incision are closed and not separated, the term used is *approximated. Clean, dry*, and *intact* are terms used to describe the dressing covering an incision. If there is any type of organ protrusion through the dehisced incision, the term used is *evisceration.*

27. B) Apply oxygen.

A patient who has overdosed on an opioid needs immediate intervention. In order of importance: Apply oxygen, administer naloxone (Narcan), and call the rapid response team and provider. Holding the next dose of pain medication would be appropriate, as would be checking with the provider for a different medication, but only after the patient has stabilized.

28. D) Vomiting, firm distended abdomen, denies flatus.

Postoperative ileus is an interruption in gastrointestinal motility. Symptoms include hypoactive or absent bowel sounds accompanied by lack of flatus; nausea and vomiting, especially with oral intake; and distended abdomen. These symptoms occur as the stomach fills with either oral intake or gastric secretions. Abdominal rigidity, increased pain, and hypoactive bowel tones could indicate bleeding. Acid reflux, active bowel tones, and passing flatus are assessment data that would not cause concern. Nausea, abdominal tenderness, and soft palpation are assessment data that fall within defined postoperative limits.

29. D) The teach-back method.

The teach-back method is used to validate a patient's understanding of information provided by asking them to retell it in their own words. It allows the provider to gauge the patient's understanding of the material and clarify any areas of need. A written questionnaire is generally used to obtain information from a patient. Closed-ended questions limit responses by eliciting yes, no, or short answers from the patient, and their value may be limited in understanding whether teaching requires clarification. A patient interview is used to obtain subjective information from the patient, not validate information provided.

30. C) Recognizes pills by appearance rather than label.

When a patient identifies pills only by appearance it is a sign of low health literacy, which should be further investigated. This can indicate an inability to read well or difficulty understanding written instruction. It is also dangerous because pills vary in appearance by manufacturer, dose, and other factors. Asking questions of the care team is a positive sign; not asking questions, on the other hand, may indicate lack of engagement or difficulty comprehending information. Bringing a care partner to appointments provides support and a second person who can digest the information provided, it is not a sign of low health literacy. Missing appointments without advance notice can be a red flag for low health literacy because it could suggest the patient is unable to understand their appointment details or has difficulty managing appointments. However, the nurse should not be immediately concerned if the patient occasionally reschedules an appointment.

31. B) Plain language.

Plain language is used to provide clear, concise, easy-to-understand information free of jargon. Complex language is the opposite of simple, plain language and should be avoided. Medical shorthand is used in writing to abbreviate medical terminology. It is not to be used when communicating with patients. Slang may be specific to certain groups or subcultures; it may not adequately convey the necessary information to all patients.

32. B) "The percutaneous drain in your abdomen should remain in place for approximately 7 days to prevent postsurgical complications."

The nurse should provide patient teaching using plain language, avoiding medical terminology, and use of complex words when more simple words can suffice. *Percutaneous drain, abdomen,* and *postsurgical* are all words that can be simplified for the patient. The nurse uses plain language by substituting the word *cuts* for *surgical incisions, belly* for *abdomen,* and *tube* for *percutaneous drain.* Straightforward communication that clearly states when a patient should take their medicine is also an example of using plain language.

33. D) Health literacy.

Health literacy is the ability to comprehend basic health information and use it to make one's own health decisions. Compliance is following directions or instructions and is often used by the healthcare team to gauge a patient's health literacy. Comprehension is one's ability to understand something and is a general term not limited to healthcare information. Cultural competence indicates one's ability to understand and appropriately interact with other cultures.

34. A) "I will just do what my spouse tells me to do."
The patient who states they will just do what their spouse tells them to do may be indicating a lack of understanding of what is expected of them. They are deferring responsibility to another person for their own healthcare determination. This should be investigated because it may indicate low health literacy. The patient who verbalizes how to take their thyroid medication repeats a clear instruction and mentions using the medication bottle as a reference for instruction. The patient who asks for a moment to write something down is showing engagement and initiative to make notes to reference later. The patient who clarifies their appointment details demonstrates engagement. If they did not show up for their appointment, further investigation may be indicated.

35. B) "I'd like to review these questions with you."
Not completing forms in their entirety is a red flag for low health literacy. Offering to go through the questions together is a nonjudgmental way to address the missing information, and it allows the nurse to assess and address any barriers that led to the patient not completing the form. Filing the incomplete form does not help the nurse gain the missing information or assess the patient's health literacy and barriers for future intervention. Asking the patient why they did not complete the form correctly is condescending and can immediately compromise the nurse–patient relationship. Although explaining the purpose of the form is appropriate, telling the patient to complete a form they already turned in does not assess or address any barriers to learning.

36. D) "Will you teach me how you will choose your foods to help manage your blood sugar? Let's start with breakfast as an example."
Asking the patient to explain the information in their own words and provide examples showing they understand the content is a form of the teach-back method. This method is preferred to closed-ended questions, which are not as effective in determining whether clarification is required. Asking whether the spouse can make adjustments is a closed-ended question. Providing a patient with written material is a good practice to support teaching, but it does not validate the patient's comprehension of the material. Asking the patient whether they are going to avoid waffles and syrup is another closed-ended question, and it may elicit a guilt response due to its judgmental nature.

37. B) Handwashing
Appropriate hand hygiene is the best way to prevent infection and is part of the aseptic technique that patients should be taught to manage drains safely. Closing the drains after emptying helps ensure adequate suction and reduces the risk of contaminants entering the drain, but it is not the primary way to reduce the risk of infection. Stripping the drains before emptying helps eliminate flow restrictions (e.g., from clots), but it does not prevent infections. Using a new measuring cup each time is preferred practice, but cleaning the measuring cup between uses is also acceptable.

38. C) Turning, coughing, and deep breathing.
To address atelectasis following surgery and reduce the risk for pneumonia, the nurse should teach all postoperative patients respiratory hygiene measures, including turning, coughing, and deep breathing. Breathing treatments may be useful in some patients postoperatively if there is impaired gas exchange or development of respiratory complications; however, they are not applicable to all postoperative patients as a basic intervention for prevention of atelectasis and pneumonia. Maintaining nothing-by-mouth status is not a respiratory intervention and is not indicated for every postoperative patient. Wearing supplemental oxygen helps to maintain oxygen levels postoperatively as needed, but it is not related to respiratory hygiene.

39. D) Postural hypotension.
Older adults are at higher risk for postural hypotension postoperatively; thus, they should be taught to change positions slowly to reduce the risks associated with postural hypotension, such as dizziness, syncope, and potential for falls. Delirium is not a normal postoperative response in older adults, and older adults are not more prone to postoperative electrolyte imbalances or pain. Additionally, although postoperative pain might be worsened by sudden changes in position, position changes are not associated with delirium or electrolyte imbalances.

40. B) Impaired wound healing.
Smoking reduces the ability of the circulatory system to carry oxygen to the tissues; therefore, impaired wound healing is a risk of smoking postoperatively. Smoking cessation has no correlation with increased risk of falls, postoperative pain levels, or postural hypotension.

41. A) Ambulation.
Practicing early ambulation post surgery promotes the return of bowel function. Drain maintenance may be an important part of postoperative care for some patients, but it has no bearing on return of normal bowel function. Maintaining nothing-by-mouth status does not promote the return of bowel function, although patients should follow the surgeon's instructions regarding timing of and advancement of diet restrictions. Postoperative incentive spirometry is best practice for improving atelectasis and reducing the risk of respiratory complications such as pneumonia.

42. B) "I keep my heating pad on my feet at night because it is cold in the house."
Patients with diabetes are at risk for peripheral neuropathy, which may limit the ability to detect dangerous temperatures in affected body parts. For this reason, patients with diabetes should be taught to avoid applying heat sources directly to the feet. Diabetes also presents the risk for impaired wound healing, so proper foot care includes reducing risk for injury either by filing the toenails instead of cutting them or by cutting the nails along the shape of the toe and then filing the sharp edges. The patient who prefers socks that reduce sweating is appropriately voicing the need to keep the feet as clean and dry as possible. Moisture increases friction, bacteria, and the potential for skin breakdown. Patients with diabetes sometimes experience the dawn phenomenon, which is increased blood sugar in the morning. Patients can help stabilize their morning glucose readings by reducing carbohydrate intake and increasing protein intake at breakfast.

43. D) Written instructions.
Written discharge instructions should be provided to all patients as part of a thorough discharge plan. This gives the patient a written reference for use when they leave the hospital in case they need reinforcement of the plan and instructions. Not all patients need a home health referral, and nurses should use such resources appropriately. The nurse has verified understanding, and the patient and caregiver expressed confidence in performing care independently, so a home health referral is not indicated. Returning belongings is best practice; however, it is not part of discharge teaching. Discharge medications are not typically provided, although the nurse should ensure that the appropriate prescriptions are either given to the patient or sent to the pharmacy.

44. B) Chewing gum.
Chewing gum is an evidence-based nonpharmacologic intervention to promote gut motility and return of bowel function, which reduces the risk of postoperative ileus. Aromatherapy and meditation are complementary therapies that can aid with pain control or reduce nausea, but evidence does not support that they promote the return of bowel function and help prevent ileus. Incentive spirometers are an important nonpharmacologic intervention for prevention of respiratory complications, not ileus.

45. D) Wound dehiscence.
Patients who have diabetes have a high risk of wound dehiscence. Additionally, smoking impairs oxygenation of the healing tissues, which can impair wound healing, further contributing to wound dehiscence. Patients with open abdominal incisions are at risk for ileus, but having diabetes and being a smoker do not directly increase the risk of developing postoperative ileus. Diabetes places the patient at risk of low blood sugar, but smoking does not impact this risk. The patient's risk factors do not directly impact the risk for postsurgical pain.

46. D) Transcutaneous electrical nerve stimulation unit.
A transcutaneous electrical nerve stimulation unit is a device that uses small electrodes attached to a stimulator to impede pain indicators when placed externally around the site of pain. It is a noninvasive, nonpharmacologic treatment that is effective for some patients. Electroconvulsive therapy is the external use of electrical stimulation to the head to treat severe depression, not pain. An intrathecal pain pump is an implanted device to deliver pain medication to the spinal fluid, not electrical stimulation. A spinal cord stimulator is implanted within the epidural space and delivers electrical impulses to the surrounding nerves. It is not noninvasive.

47. B) Offer to turn on the patient's favorite music.
Music or calming sounds can help ease the agitated or confused patient without the use of medications and should be offered as a complementary therapy. Light massage can be used for agitated patients who are not violent. With this patient's recent violent episodes, it is best to try another alternative therapy that does not involve touch, especially without asking the patient first. Calling security or using restraints can escalate the patient's behavior and do nothing to calm or reassure them.

48. A) "I am going to help you get up and take a walk around the unit."

The nurse who initiates getting the patient out of bed is promoting early ambulation, which is evidence-based practice to help reduce the risks of ileus, thrombus, atelectasis, and pneumonia. Pain management and control of pain before it becomes intolerable is best practice but does not prevent ileus, thrombus, atelectasis, and pneumonia. Wearing sequential compression devices on the legs while immobile is a best practice intervention for preventing thrombus formation but does not promote the prevention of ileus, atelectasis, or pneumonia. Using the incentive spirometer 10 times/hr while awake can help reduce atelectasis and pneumonia risk but does not address ileus and thrombus formation.

49. A) Try to find a relaxation or meditation video on the hospital's TV system.

The patient is voicing that the pain is more discomfort and nagging pain, not uncontrolled pain. Complementary therapies work in conjunction with opioid pain medication to provide pain management and comfort measures. These should be a first-line intervention to promote comfort and relaxation for the patient who does not want to take more medications. The patient already stated that they did not want more opioid pain medication, and the nurse should respect their wishes and not push a therapy the patient does not want. The nurse should try other interventions, such as nonpharmacologic therapies, before calling the provider; further, the patient does not want something stronger for their pain, so the nurse would not be respecting the patient's wishes by requesting stronger pain medication from the provider. Giving a medication for reasons other than those on the order/MAR is operating outside of the nurse's scope and is not appropriate. The nurse would need to contact the provider for a change to the ibuprofen (Advil) parameters if there is a need to use it for pain or any other reason but fever.

50. B) Aromatherapy.

Aromatherapy is an evidence-based nonpharmacologic treatment that can be combined with both pain medication and antiemetic use for pain and nausea reduction. The use of abdominal binders can help reduce postsurgical pain, especially during mobility, but it is not a complementary therapy for nausea. Light-box therapy is useful for patients with depression or sundowning. Muscle relaxants, which can be combined with opioid pain management for pain control, are pharmacologic treatments.

51. A) Call the provider and request an alternative medication for the patient's pain.

Meperidine (Demerol) is a high-risk medication for older patients due to the effects on metabolic processes and seizure risk. It should be avoided if there are alternatives that can be used. It is best to advocate for the patient and call the provider for an alternative pain medication that can be given with less risk to the patient with severe pain. It is not appropriate to give the meperidine (Demerol) without first advocating for the patient due to the risks for older patients. Also, it is not appropriate to disregard the NPO order and give the PO hydrocodone/acetaminophen (Norco). The hydrocodone/acetaminophen (Norco) is also ordered for pain of 4-7, and the patient reports pain of 8 out of 10, so it is not indicated per the provider's order. Offering alternative therapies is best used in conjunction with analgesic pain medication, especially in the setting of severe pain. Music can be offered to the patient, but the nurse should not just choose music to play without discussing it with the patient first. It is also not the first-line intervention to get the patient's pain under control.

52. C) Offer to assist the patient with breathing exercises during the dressing change.
Diversional activities, such as focused breathing, music, or meditation, can help the patient handle acute pain associated with dressing changes or painful interventions. Diversional therapies can also be useful to calm a patient who is fearful or anxious. This is the appropriate first-line intervention. Asking the wound care nurse to come back is not an ideal intervention, as the patient is not refusing to participate. Supporting the patient with diversional activities is a better solution than delaying the therapy. The patient is not reporting increased pain at this time but is voicing fearfulness and anxiety around the unfamiliar procedure. Asking the provider for more pain medicine is not appropriate unless the patient should voice an increase in pain or the inability to tolerate the procedure. Telling the patient the procedure will be quick and others do fine with it invalidates the patient's fears and can harm the nurse–patient relationship.

53. A) Bleeding.
Naproxen is a nonsteroidal anti-inflammatory drug (NSAID), and the most common side effects of NSAID use are gastrointestinal irritation, ulcers, and bleeding. Body aches are not a common side effect of NSAID use. Constipation is associated with opioid pain medication, not NSAIDs. Cough is sometimes associated with angiotensin-converting enzyme (ACE) inhibitors but is not a common side effect of NSAID use.

54. B) H_2 receptor agonists
H_2 receptor agonists (H_2 blockers) should be added to protect the gastrointestinal system from side effects of NSAIDs such as irritation, ulceration, and bleeding. Calcium channel blockers are used to lower blood pressure and do not protect against gastrointestinal symptoms associated with NSAID use. Laxatives are used to treat constipation and do not alleviate the negative gastrointestinal symptoms associated with NSAID use. Opioids are used to treat pain and do not provide gastrointestinal protection.

55. C) Constipation
Constipation is a common side effect of opioid medication use. Steps to reduce the risk of constipation include ambulation, increased fluid intake, increased fiber intake, and use of stool softeners or laxatives. Appropriate use of pain medication reduces the risk of dependency on opioids. Allergic reactions, although they can occur with any medication, are not improved with ambulation, diet, or fluid intake changes. Diarrhea is not associated with opioid use, which often causes constipation.

56. A) "Avoid drinking grapefruit juice."
Grapefruit juice is contraindicated with statin use, including simvastatin (Lipitor) for high cholesterol. It decreases the metabolism of the drug, causing it to be stronger than indicated, leading to toxicity. Statins are not meant for as-needed use but for daily use. It is not necessary to take statins on an empty stomach. Taking statins alone is not reliable to "fix" high cholesterol. This medication should be used in conjunction with diet modification and exercise.

57. C) The patient's diet.

Vitamin K–containing foods can interfere with the patient's achievement of therapeutic INR and subsequent drug dosing during warfarin (Coumadin) therapy. The nurse should investigate the patient's diet, specifically vitamin K–rich foods, and find out whether the patient's intake of such foods has fluctuated in the last month or since starting warfarin therapy. The patient's physical activity and sleep patterns do not affect therapeutic levels of warfarin. Consumption of certain fruit juices, such as grapefruit and cranberry, should be investigated as they have an effect on warfarin therapy. However, orange juice intake is not a cause for concern.

58. A) Actively listening.

Active listening is an example of a therapeutic communication technique the nurse can use during the conversation and is appropriate to use when the patient shares personal information. Continuing to ask questions that ignore what the patient is saying can be insensitive. Referring the patient to a mental health counselor can be appropriate later, but not in the moment. Using humor to lighten the mood may not be appropriate in this situation if the nurse has not built a rapport with the patient.

59. D) Working with the parents and patient to set specific goals based on their needs.

Involving the patient and their parents in the process is important to ensure all needs are met. Working with just the parents excludes the patient as an active participant in their care. Goal setting with just the patient is not appropriate because the patient is a minor with an intellectual/developmental disability. Telling the parents there is a plan is not enough because this does not encourage active participation in the care process.

60. D) Silence.

Silence is when the nurse does not talk but allows the patient time to reflect on what has been said. Clarification is when further questions are answered to gain a better understanding. Informing is when the nurse provides information. Restating occurs when the nurse repeats back to the patient what was said.

61. B) Explaining the risks associated with herbal remedy use and possible drug interactions

The nurse would demonstrate culturally competent care by providing education to the patient about the risks associated with using herbal remedies and any drug interactions involved with the use of specific herbs. Undermining the patients' beliefs about their health would be culturally insensitive. Although it is important to notify the provider, this would not be an immediate nurse-led action. Taking the herbal remedies away is not appropriate because they are the patient's property.

62. C) Ask the patient more questions about their spiritual needs and refer them to the chaplain if the patient agrees.
Asking the patient additional questions will help the nurse understand how important the patient's spiritual/religious beliefs are to them and how they affect their beliefs about health and healing. Chaplains are typically trained to help meet the spiritual needs of all patients. Telling the patient not to worry and that they are in good hands in the hospital, then continuing with the health history, is not a therapeutic response because it diminishes the patient's feelings and does not address their spiritual needs. Nurses should not make assumptions about patients. The patient has not expressed being Christian, so offering a bible is not appropriate. The patient may practice a different religion or no religion at all and still consider themself to be spiritual. For many people, their spiritual beliefs are intertwined with their beliefs about health, and it is insensitive for the nurse to ignore the patients' spiritual needs.

63. B) "Can you tell me more about what you are hoping for with this new plan of care?"
It is important to use open-ended questions when assessing a patient's goals of care and when communicating about palliative care because this can be a very difficult and emotional decision for a patient and their family. "Can you tell me more about what you are hoping for with this new plan of care?" is an open-ended question that allows for further communication. Closed-ended questions that elicit only yes or no responses will not provide the nurse with the information needed to accurately assess the patient. They also will not help strengthen the nurse–patient relationship. "Are you sure you don't want to continue treatment?"; "Did the doctor talk to you about your illness?"; and "Do you want to stay at home?" are all closed-ended questions.

64. A) Posttraumatic stress disorder.
Individuals with prior military service may have been exposed to violent or traumatic events that can place them at higher risk for posttraumatic stress disorder. Experience in the military does not significantly impact one's risk of developing cardiovascular disease, hypertension, or hyperlipidemia when compared with the general population.

65. A) Annual mammograms.
There are three types of prevention in healthcare: primary, secondary, and tertiary. Secondary prevention involves measures to minimize the impact of illness or injury that is already present. It includes such things as mammograms, screenings, and lab tests to identify existing health issues in their earliest stages. Primary prevention involves active measures to avoid illness or injury. Handwashing, immunizations, dedicated personal items, and standard precautions are all considered primary prevention. Tertiary prevention aims to mitigate the effects of health issues that are more advanced. Examples include physical or occupational rehabilitation to help patients live with chronic disorders.

66. B) Artificial passive

Immunity is the body's ability to ward off infection by means of antibodies. Antibodies are acquired both naturally and artificially. Passive artificial immunity would occur in a patient receiving a blood transfusion that contains antibodies. Active artificial immunity occurs through means of a vaccination, through which the attenuated antigens are introduced to the body in order to stimulate antibody production. Active natural immunity occurs when a person's immune system is attacked by antigens. The body builds a defense of antibodies in response. Passive natural immunity occurs in instances of antibodies being passed to infants via breastmilk.

67. B) Congenital heart defect.

Nonmodifiable risk factors include such conditions as congenital heart defects, hereditary diseases, and autoimmune disorders. Modifiable risk factors are those that can be decreased or prevented by changes in habits. Smoking, diet, and exercise are the most common modifiable risk factors in heart disease.

68. B) Ensure it is safe to administer specific vaccines by checking with the provider.

The patient receiving chemotherapy is immunocompromised. It is important for these patients to be protected with vaccines safely, so the nurse must check with the primary care provider first to ensure appropriate vaccine choice. Live virus vaccines must be avoided in immunocompromised patients. The nurse should not choose appropriate vaccines alone, but should collaborate with the primary care provider to ensure safety of vaccine choice. It is not appropriate for the nurse to provide all vaccines available without first checking with the patient's primary care provider for safety and specific vaccine choice. Most vaccines are deferred while a patient is actively receiving chemotherapy; however, not all vaccines must be avoided. For example, patients in active chemotherapy treatment are encouraged to receive a flu vaccine.

69. A) Autosomal dominant.

Autosomal dominant disorders are those passed through a single gene. Autosomal recessive inheritance requires the trait to be on two genes to present. *Complex recessive* refers to inheritance of disorders that cause problems with cellular regulation. Sex-linked recessive disorders or diseases are those present only on the X or Y chromosomes.

70. A) "Have you received the bacille Calmette–Guérin (BCG) vaccine in the past?"

Patients who have received the BCG vaccine in the past will have a skin test reaction that typically wanes in intensity over the years. These patients should be further evaluated with chest x-ray or other diagnostic tests in the setting of inconclusive skin test results. The nurse should not notify the health department at this time, as they have not appropriately assessed and verified a positive TB diagnosis. The nurse cannot determine that the patient is TB positive by visual inspection of the skin test. Appropriate reading of the skin test involves measuring the raised area (area of induration), not the redness, and determining the patient's risk level. The nurse should then notify the provider for further orders. The nurse stating that the "red bump is pretty small, so I think its fine" does not appropriately assess the site by measuring the induration and assessing the patient's risk level.

71. C) Complete a nutrition screening tool and contact the registered dietician per facility protocol.
Interdisciplinary collaboration for patients with suspected malnutrition, no matter the cause, is the most comprehensive way to appropriately address the patient's nutrition state. The patient shows signs of dehydration (skin tenting) and malnutrition (brittle hair/nails and muscle wasting), so further intervention is warranted. A screening tool gives the interdisciplinary team information on which to base their assessment, and the registered dietician is a resource to provide interventions appropriate for the patient's nutritional needs. The patient is NPO for a clear reason, as delaying tests can delay potential surgical interventions. It is appropriate to call the provider for intravenous fluid therapy initiation if none is ordered at this time and the patient is to remain NPO. Further screenings and investigation are indicated based on the patient's inability to provide a reliable history. Calling the facility and/or family for a report of the patient's nutritional history and physical capabilities would help provide a more thorough picture of the patient's nutritional needs as well as the care they are receiving and should certainly be done; however, the nurse has no basis to suspect mistreatment, and making that accusation would be irresponsible and unethical. Signs of dehydration and malnutrition are not a normal part of the aging process. Assuming this and doing nothing when further intervention is appropriate is not best practice.

72. C) Exercise regimen.
Simvastatin (Zocor) is prescribed for high cholesterol. Managing high cholesterol is best achieved through diet, exercise, and a medication plan. Simvastatin (Zocor) prescribed for high cholesterol should not be confused with sertraline (Zoloft) for depression or other psychologic conditions. There is no indication the patient needs depression education or resources at this time. Simvastatin is not prescribed for diabetes, and there is no indication that the patient has diabetes. A low-residue diet is low in fiber content and is indicated for certain gastrointestinal disorders or procedures.

73. C) Smoking cessation.
The patient has several risk factors for cardiovascular disease, including hypertension, high cholesterol, diabetes, and smoking. The nurse recognizes that smoking cessation is a modifiable factor that can reduce the patient's risk. There is no indication that the patient needs a calcium-rich diet. Thyroid function and calcium levels are interdependent, but there is no evidence that the patient needs this intervention. There is also no indication that the patient should increase their fiber intake without further assessment. The patient has not indicated that they have a high-stress lifestyle, so further assessment is needed to determine whether this is a necessary education topic for this patient.

74. C) Monitor and document vital signs.
Overall vital signs comparison during the first 15 minutes of transfusion allows the nurse to monitor for indicators of a blood transfusion reaction. The patient's energy level would not immediately increase as the blood is transfusing, nor would the hemoglobin until the unit of blood has been administered. The provider typically orders a repeat hemoglobin blood level after the entire unit of blood has infused. Urine output is insignificant in the early part of the transfusion.

75. A) Antibiotics

Clostridium difficile infection is an adverse effect of antibiotic therapy, with symptoms including frequent, watery stools; abdominal pain; bloating; and nausea. Antibiotic use alters the normal gut bacteria, which allows for overgrowth of *C. difficile* and subsequent infection in some patients. Diuretics for water excretion, antiemetics for nausea, and beta blockers for hypertension do not increase the risk of *C. difficile* infection.

76. B) Constipation.

Constipation is common in older adults and is directly related to a patient's nutrition and hydration status, medication usage, and level of activity or mobility. Osteoarthritis can impact mobility, and many patients with the condition use medications to treat it; however, neither mobility nor medication usage is a cause of osteoarthritis. Similarly, nutrition and hydration status are not risk factors. Taste buds decrease in quantity and sensitivity over time, causing some older adults to experience loss of taste. Loss of taste can also be a side effect of some medications. Assessment of the patient's nutrition and hydration status and medications may help the nurse assess for this complication, but loss of taste is not related to a patient's mobility. Hearing loss, a common complication of aging, is not related to a patient's nutrition or hydration status or mobility.

77. A) Conflict of interest.

This situation presents a conflict of interest because the nurses are being incentivized to promote a particular medication to patients. Nurses should identify and avoid conflicts of interest at all costs. The nurses would be promoting use of the medication based on personal gain rather than on validated data, which does not follow evidence-based practice. Recommending this medication based on an incentive could be harmful to patients, and it is outside of the scope of the nurse's role; patient advocacy is acting on the patient's behalf. Interprofessional collaboration would involve working with other disciplines to provide patient care.

78. A) Calcium carbonate (Tums) and calcitriol (Rocaltrol).

Perioral numbness or tingling, as well as tingling of the distal extremities, is an early sign of hypocalcemia, a potential complication from thyroid surgery. This occurs due to temporary or permanent damage done to the parathyroid glands during thyroid surgery. To treat hypocalcemia, depending on lab values, the nurse should anticipate administering a combination of oral or intravenous calcium (calcium carbonate or calcium gluconate) and calcitriol (Rocaltrol), a form of activated vitamin D, which aids in the absorption of calcium until the parathyroid glands regain function to regulate the serum calcium. Ibuprofen (Advil) and gabapentin (Neurontin) are often given postoperatively as a multimodal approach to pain management. The patient reports a low pain score, which does not indicate a necessary intervention. Lisinopril (Prinivil) and hydrochlorothiazide (Microzide) are administered to treat high blood pressure; the patient's blood pressure is within normal parameters and does not require intervention. Oxycodone acetaminophen (Percocet) and docusate sodium (Colace) may be prescribed postoperatively for pain and constipation. The patient is reporting a low pain score and voices no other concerns, such as constipation, which means that this medication combination is not an appropriate choice.

79. A) Assess whether risk of injury by not using restraints is greater than risk of using restraints.
Physical restraints present physical and emotional risks for patients. To decide whether their use is warranted, the nurse must first assess whether the risk they pose is less than the risk they are meant to prevent. After determining that the risk is less with restraint use, the nurse should obtain an order from the provider, notify the patient's family of the restraint use, and determine whether the hospital has the appropriate type of restraints in stock.

80. C) Magnesium 1.2 mg/dL (0.49 mmol/L).
The magnesium has most likely been depleted due to severe diarrhea because it is absorbed in the small intestine and excreted in stool. Magnesium is vital for neuromuscular function. Low magnesium contributes to EKG changes, including PVCs. The patient's blood glucose is within normal limits. The patient's hemoglobin is slightly decreased, but this would not cause cardiac issues. Sodium is decreased, as would be expected due to diarrhea, but decreased sodium would not cause cardiac issues.

81. B) Facial nerve, cranial nerve VII.
Bell's palsy is a typically temporary condition characterized by weakened or paralyzed muscles on one side of the face. It is caused by dysfunction or inflammation surrounding the facial nerve (cranial nerve VII), which controls the facial muscles, allowing for movement and expression of the face. The other cranial nerves are not involved in facial movement. The accessory nerve (cranial nerve XI) controls muscles of the neck, which control turning the head and elevating the shoulders. The glossopharyngeal nerve (cranial nerve IX) controls swallowing and taste. The trochlear nerve (cranial nerve IV) runs to the superior oblique muscle of the eye and helps control eye movement.

82. B) "Will you receive blood products if you need a blood transfusion?"
If a patient has a known bleed and hemoglobin is low, the patient may need a blood transfusion. The nurse must understand the patient's wishes about receiving blood products, which may be an emergent need. It is important for the healthcare team to know whether the patient agrees to receive blood products as a practicing Jehovah's Witness because this religion prohibits administration of blood products. When the patient last urinated is not relevant information for this situation, and inquiring about a spiritual advisor visit or a drink preference is not applicable to the diagnosis.

83. A) Constipation.
Chronic use of opioids, such as tramadol, poses a risk of constipation. Opioid use is not a risk factor for diabetes, peripheral vascular disease, or pneumonia. Diabetes mellitus is insulin resistance. It is affected by genetic factors as well as by diet and physical activity. Peripheral vascular disease is caused by plaque buildup within arterial walls, which limits blood flow to extremities. Pneumonia is an infectious process caused by a bacteria, virus, or fungus.

84. B) Metformin (Glucophage)

Metformin (Glucophage) should be stopped 24 hours before any iodine contrast studies, and restart should be delayed for at least 48 hours after the test due to risk of lactic acidosis. Levothyroxine (Synthroid) is a synthetic thyroid hormone used for thyroid hormone replacement and is not contraindicated in contrast studies. Polyethylene glycol (Miralax) is a laxative that helps pull or retain water in the bowels and evacuate them. It is not contraindicated for contrast studies. Prednisolone (Omnipred) is a steroid used to reduce inflammation and is not contraindicated for contrast studies.

85. A) Angiotensin-converting enzyme (ACE) inhibitor.

A dry, troublesome cough is a side effect of ACE inhibitors and angiotensin receptor blockers (ARBs) used to treat high blood pressure, of which the patient reports having a history. Antacids, also used to treat reflux, are not known to cause a dry, irritating cough. A dry, nagging cough is not a side effect of diuretics, which may be used to treat high blood pressure or fluid retention caused by other disease processes, such as heart failure. PPIs are used to treat GERD but are not commonly known to cause a dry, troublesome cough.

86. C) Erythematous rash covering the face and neck

An erythematous rash covering the face and neck could indicate a hypersensitivity reaction, also known as *red man syndrome*. The nurse should discontinue the infusion, assess the patient's level of stability, and contact the provider. Allergy to azithromycin (Zithromax) 500 mg is not concerning as there is no cross-sensitivity link between vancomycin (Vancocin) and azithromycin; administering a vancomycin infusion to a patient with an azithromycin allergy is safe. Audible crackles in the right lung base is an expected finding of community-acquired pneumonia. Although the white blood cell count is elevated, this is an expected finding in an individual who has community-acquired pneumonia.

87. A) Assess the serum creatinine level.

Vancomycin (Vancocin) may result in nephrotoxicity and renal failure; therefore, the priority nursing assessment is to review the patient's creatinine level prior to administering an intravenous vancomycin infusion. Although the nurse should assess the right lower extremity pulses and document the findings as part of the comprehensive assessment, it is not the priority assessment before starting the vancomycin infusion. Use of antibiotics may increase the risk of developing *Clostridium difficile;* however, it is not a priority for the nurse to obtain an occult stool sample before administering vancomycin. The nurse should assess the white blood cell count later, to evaluate the patient's response to treatment.

88. C) Metformin (Glucophage) ER 500 mg by mouth at bedtime.

Cardiac catheterization is a procedure that uses contrast dye and x-ray imaging to view the coronary vessels. Studies have found that the use of contrast dye in patients taking metformin can cause lactic acidosis. The nurse should notify the provider that the patient is taking metformin (Glucophage) ER 500 mg by mouth at bedtime. There are no contraindications related to the use of contrast dye in patients taking amlodipine (Norvasc), atorvastatin (Lipitor), or fish oil. Amlodipine 5 mg by mouth daily can be prescribed for the treatment of hypertension. Amlodipine has a renal protective effect. This patient has a history of hyperlipidemia, which explains the use of atorvastatin. Fish oil is used as an adjunct treatment for hyperlipidemia.

89. D) Risk for ineffective peripheral perfusion.

Peripheral tissue perfusion is the priority in the instance of a wrist fracture because adding oxygenated blood to the fracture is vital for the healing process. When there is a fracture, inflammation and swelling increase the risk for blood clots in that area. The edema can also impede adequate blood flow. Impaired mobility is a more likely diagnosis for fracture of a lower extremity, and even then it would likely pose a lower risk than inadequate perfusion. *Risk for disuse syndrome* refers to the loss of ability to adequately use a body part such as an appendage; healing of the fracture is unlikely to disrupt use long-term. Although the patient may experience acute pain related to the fracture, it is unlikely to pose a risk to the patient.

90. B) Risk for impaired tissue perfusion.

When a patient is immobile, prolonged pressure to the skin can impede blood circulation. When blood flow is impeded long enough, the cells in the area and surrounding areas are deprived of adequate oxygen. Maintaining good perfusion to all areas of the body is vital. Acute confusion is a sudden change in cognition and often points to a larger medical problem. Although the patient's statement may indicate a need for education regarding the purpose of the interventions, the patient is alert and oriented, so the nursing diagnosis of acute confusion would be inappropriate. Toileting self-care deficit occurs when a patient who can ambulate is unable to reach the bathroom in time. *Impaired bed mobility* refers to the loss of ability to self-mobilize. In this case, tissue perfusion is the priority.

91. B) Bowel obstruction

A bowel obstruction is the absence of gastric motility. Therefore, the nursing diagnosis of dysfunctional gastrointestinal motility would be appropriate. Appendicitis does not directly cause impaired gastrointestinal motility. Gallstones cause severe pain but do not affect the motility of the gastrointestinal tract. *Diarrhea* refers to the overly motile bowel and the stool produced.

92. D) Repeat serum sodium levels.

The patient is experiencing hyponatremia with a sodium level of 125 mEq/L. It is crucial for the nurse to assess repeat sodium levels because if the sodium level corrects too rapidly, with a greater than 8 to 12 mEq/L increase in the first 24 hours, it can cause osmotic demyelination syndrome, which can lead to life-threatening seizures and coma. The nurse may still assess lung sounds to monitor for fluid overload, but monitoring sodium levels can help to avoid potentially irreversible harm. Reviewing the patient's dietary intake of sodium should happen after the patient's sodium level is restored to normal. The nurse will need to monitor neurologic status if the sodium levels rise too rapidly.

93. D) Risk for unstable blood glucose.

Steroids, while decreasing inflammation, often cause increased blood glucose levels. Glucose levels will need to be monitored and managed. Monitoring glucose levels well and managing them can prevent elevated glucose levels. Imbalanced nutrition is related to poor dietary intake; this patient's blood sugar elevation is associated with medication use, not diet. Electrolyte imbalances do not directly relate to steroid treatments or glucose levels. Addressing the glucose levels early and monitoring them can prevent metabolic imbalance from developing.

94. B) Administer the scheduled dose.

The nurse would administer the scheduled dose and recheck the patient's pulse in 30 minutes. If the pulse is still high, the nurse can then administer the PRN IV dose. The nurse should administer only one dose at a time and perform the assessment before administering a second dose. The nurse would not need to clarify the order and only needs to contact the provider if both the scheduled dose and the PRN dose are ineffective. The nurse should use all interventions and evaluate outcomes before calling for new orders. The nurse would not hold metoprolol without a provider's order.

95. C) Patient grimacing and tense, pulse rate 105 bpm, rates pain 6/10.

A patient who is grimacing and tense, has an elevated pulse rate, and rates pain above 5/10 is showing signs that the dose administered was not effective enough to give relief. A patient will often demonstrate nonverbal signs of pain (e.g., grimacing) as well as physiologic signs. Taking both subjective and objective data into consideration is important when monitoring the effectiveness of pain medication. Ambulating and a 5/10 rating shows effective pain control, although a rating above 5/10 could warrant additional pain relief measures. Although a sleeping patient may not present subjective signs of pain, it is important to ask patients to rate their pain when possible.

96. D) 80 mL of sanguineous drainage

Sanguineous drainage is essentially bleeding. Emptying a large amount of blood from a drain is cause for concern. A small amount of serous drainage is to be expected with drain output in many cases. Often serous drainage is seen in instances in which large amounts of washout were used during surgery. The drain has been placed because of the abscess; purulent drainage is expected in this instance and would not be cause for concern. Serosanguineous drainage is to be expected with many drains as well; often it is an indication of a healthy incision.

97. D) Wait for an interpreter from the facility's language service department.

Only staff who are validated interpreters or an approved video interpreter service are acceptable to use to interpret; therefore, the nurse must wait for the language service department to provide an interpreter. The nurse should avoid having another floor nurse who speaks the same language assist unless they have been validated as an interpreter. The use of family and friends should also be avoided due to patient confidentiality issues and the risk of bias or of personal understanding of the information being miscommunicated. If the patient requests that their loved one interpret, the nurse should respect this request only if an approved interpreter is present to validate the information being communicated.

98. A) Administration of nitroglycerin (Nitrolingual)

The patient is exhibiting symptoms of a heart attack, in which case a vasodilator, such as nitroglycerin (Nitrolingual), may be indicated. However, the patient has taken sildenafil (Viagra), which is also a vasodilator. These medications are contraindicated together due to the potential for a dangerous drop in blood pressure. Drawing the patient's labs, initiating oxygen therapy, and administering IV fluids are all appropriate interventions and are not contraindicated by any of the patient's symptoms or recent intake.

99. D) Picture board.

A picture board with easy-to-recognize symbols that the patient can point to helps facilitate communication with some patients with dementia. A braille board is an assistive device for patients who are blind and can read braille; this would not aid the patient with dementia. A sound amplifier can be used for patients who are hard of hearing. The patient with dementia has difficulty with memory, not hearing loss; thus, this would not be an appropriate tool. An interpreter will not aid communication for the patient with dementia unless there is a need due to language barrier.

100. A) Introduce themself to the patient and family in the room.

Patients should be treated with dignity and respect no matter what mental state they are in. Nurses introducing themselves to both the patient and the family members is standard professional practice. The nurse should introduce themself to the patient even if the patient's mental status is altered; it is important to include the patient as much as possible and to continue to provide education and comfort. It would be unprofessional for the nurse to not introduce themself or to ignore the patient's family when entering the room.

101. C) Request medical interpreter services.

Best practice and hospital policies often require patients to be provided with medical interpreting services by a certified medical interpreter. Unless the coworker is certified as an interpreter, it is not best practice to ask for their help with translation. It is not appropriate to have a minor interpret sensitive medical information. Mobile translation applications cannot be used in place of a qualified medical interpreter.

102. B) Cultural competency

The nurse is demonstrating understanding of the importance of the patient's spirituality and beliefs, which aligns best with the nursing principle of cultural competency. These beliefs are directly related to the patient's unique cultural background. Although the nurse may also demonstrate caring, flexibility, and holistic nursing principles, it is most likely that the nurse is demonstrating cultural competence when respecting these cultural wishes.

103. A) Ask the patient which family member they want as their primary decision maker.

Advanced care planning is important, and the nurse can engage the patient in questions about who they want to make decisions for them in the event they are not able to. Continuing to allow multiple family members to make decisions may add to the confusion. However, although it is ideal for one person to be the primary decision maker, the patient, not the family, should identify that person. It is important to ensure the family understands the plan of care, but additional action is needed to avoid confusion between the family and nursing staff. It would not be appropriate for the nurse to ask the family members to stop visiting because they are the patient's support system.

104. B) Chvostek's sign.

Hypocalcemia impairs nerve conduction and muscle contractions. This can cause a variety of symptoms such as numbness and tingling of the lips or extremities, muscle spasms or twitching, seizures, and arrhythmias, depending on the severity of the hypocalcemia. Stimulating a positive Chvostek's sign indicates excitability of the facial nerve, which is an indicator of low calcium levels or hypocalcemia. Allen's test is used to determine arterial blood supply to the hand, not assess for nerve or muscle impairment, which would be indicators of hypocalcemia. This test is used to determine viability of radial arteries for harvesting in graft surgeries. The Montreal Cognitive Assessment (MoCA) checks for cognitive impairment, not for nerve or muscle weakening, and is not an indicator of hypocalcemia. It is used to assess for dementia. The Romberg test evaluates balance and coordination impairment, not muscle or nerve impairment relating to hypocalcemia. This test is beneficial in determining the root cause of ataxia (impaired coordination) and can be used for diagnosing multiple sclerosis.

105. B) Contact the surgeon; surgery may need to be postponed until the patient has abstained from alcohol.

Patients with excessive alcohol consumption are at an increased risk for complications during surgery and increased hospital stays. Because the patient drinks six beers a day, they are at high risk for injury, and the surgery might be postponed. Providing information regarding Alcoholics Anonymous is part of the patient education the nurse should offer the patient, but it is not pertinent to the immediate issue of addressing medical status for surgery. Although the patient will need to have additional laboratory tests done to assess liver function, the tests will not address the immediate surgery needs, and liver function test results will likely not impact the gallbladder surgery. Regular alcohol consumption increases risk of malnutrition, but including this diagnosis in the care plan does not address the preoperative needs.

106. A) Airway.

Airway compromise is a potentially life-threatening complication of thyroid surgery. Airway assessment and intervention always take priority in postoperative assessment of patients. Drain output, if applicable, is an important tool in assessing postoperative thyroid patients for bleeding. However, it does not take priority over the initial airway assessment. Although certain laboratory values are important to monitor for thyroid patients postoperatively, they do not take priority over assessing the airway. Pain assessment is also important for all postoperative patients; however, it is not the priority.

107. C) Privacy and confidentiality.

The nurse in this scenario understands that providing unauthorized individuals with sensitive health information is a breach of privacy and confidentiality and subject to the Health Insurance Portability and Accountability Act of 1996 (HIPAA). Advance directives are not affected. The plan of care may be affected because of the breach in privacy, but it will be an indirect effect. The patient's *right to information* refers to the right for the patient to receive information about their health and medical diagnoses; this right would not be impacted.

108. D) Refuse medical treatment.
Ultimately, the patient has the right to refuse treatment and medical services whenever they want, and this must be upheld. Hospital records are unable to be deleted or altered unless there is an error found. The patient's primary care provider might not be a staff member at the hospital, so the patient may not be able to receive care from their own provider while at the hospital. Hospitals do not hold rooms for patients who go home; if the patient goes home for the night, they will have to return as a new admission and likely to a new room.

109. D) Moral uncertainty and distress.
The nurse is trained to provide medical care and supportive services to the patient. When the patient has made a conscious decision to withdraw care, the nurse must respect that decision even if they or others disagree with it. The conflicting input from the patient's parents and/or the nurse's own opinion may cause the nurse to feel moral uncertainty and distress in this situation. The patient, rather than the nurse, may feel a lack of autonomy in this situation. Provided that the parents are involved in the patient's care and have permission to hear sensitive information, the nurse is not violating the patient's privacy rights. The nurse has not acted with dishonesty or a lack of integrity, although that may change if the nurse takes actions that support the parents' wishes over those of the patient.

110. B) "I'm sorry, but I don't think that would be appropriate."
Establishing boundaries with patients is important to maintain a therapeutic relationship. Being added to the patient's social media risks violating those boundaries, and the nurse should explain that politely. Even if the nurse doesn't have a social media account, it would be helpful to explain why the practice is not appropriate. Although some hospitals may have policies restricting this kind of practice, the most appropriate response would be to explain to the patient why the nurse cannot add them on social media.

111. A) Demonstrating respect.
The American Nurses Association's Provision 1 in the *Code of Ethics* explains that respecting patients' decisions even when the nurse does not agree with them is important in establishing a professional relationship built on trust. Detaching oneself emotionally from patients is not necessary to maintain a working relationship with the patient. Although the nurse is encouraged to keep personal opinions to themself and maintain professional rapport, that is not the best description of the support the nurse is demonstrating. Overcoming bias is not a consideration because there are no cultural, racial, or socioeconomic factors.

112. D) Report the incident to the hospital ethics committee.
The hospital ethics committee will be able to manage this situation appropriately by talking to the provider and the spouse and advocating on the patient's behalf. The patient has a right to refuse treatment, and unless the spouse has the legal right to make healthcare decisions on the patient's behalf (e.g., through power of attorney), intervention by the nurse is needed. Doing nothing is not appropriate; the nurse has a responsibility to advocate for the patient's well-being. Addressing this directly with the patient may cause conflict in the relationship between the patient and the spouse, which might lead to resentment toward the nurse and impact the therapeutic relationship. Reporting directly to the ethics committee will ensure that the issue is handled in a confidential manner.

113. B) Fluid overload.

Signs of fluid overload are an increased respiratory rate, shallow respirations, moist crackles indicating fluid in the lungs on auscultation, and shortness of breath. Although shortness of breath is associated with emphysema, it is usually also associated with activity. Patients with emphysema experience productive coughing with wheezing on auscultation, not crackles. Pleurisy, which is caused by inflammation of the lung lining and chest cavity, may also cause shortness of breath but is marked by a rubbing sound that can be heard on auscultation, not wet crackles. Tuberculosis is characterized by a persistent cough and hemoptysis or coughing up blood. Patients may also report pain in the chest due to coughing. Crackles, shallow breathing, and rapid respiratory rate are not commonly characteristic of tuberculosis.

114. C) Having a conversation with the patient about their behavior.

The patient is shouting but not displaying any signs of physical aggression. The nurse can first try to approach the patient, use therapeutic communication techniques, and establish boundaries about their behavior. Asking the provider to discharge the patient is not appropriate if the patient requires medical treatment. Delaying or refusing to provide care can cause an ethical dilemma for the nurse and place the patient at risk of a safety event. The nurse can call security if the behavior escalates and makes the nurse feel physically unsafe.

115. C) Fluid balance.

Weight is the most accurate gauge of fluid status. To ensure reliable weights, it is important to weigh the patient using the same scale and at the same time each day. Blood sugar must be measured using a small amount of blood; scale weight offers no relevant information. Although electrolytes and fluid balance are interrelated, one must use bloodwork to determine electrolyte levels. Infection is indicated in blood work and is not related to the scale.

116. C) Sodium restricted.

A sodium-restricted diet will be used for this patient due to the role of sodium in retaining water. Sodium draws water to wherever the sodium concentration is higher. Sodium is an extracellular electrolyte; thus, water is drawn out of the cells, creating water retention. Limiting sodium creates diuresis and, thus, a decrease in water retention. A low-cholesterol diet does not regulate sodium intake and impact fluid retention to aid in treatment of liver failure with ascites. Likewise, a low-fiber diet is not indicated because fiber does not contribute sodium to the diet and affect water retention. A vegetarian diet is not particularly indicated in the setting of fluid retention because it does not regulate sodium and thus water balance.

117. C) Rhabdomyolysis.

Rhabdomyolysis involves the rapid breakdown of muscle tissue, often due to severe muscle damage resulting from extreme physical activity, trauma, or burns. The rapid breakdown releases proteins called myoglobins, which can lead to acute kidney failure as evidenced by dark urine and low urine output. Other symptoms can include muscle pain or weakness. Gout, although related to kidney function, is inflammation caused by a buildup of uric acid and is not related to extreme exercise. Gout presents as pain in the joints, often affecting the big toe. Muscle atrophy is the loss of muscle mass or tone. There are various causes of muscle atrophy, but exercise does not lead to muscle atrophy, and it is not characterized by kidney failure. A urinary tract infection is caused by bacteria and is unrelated to extreme exercise.

118. A) Apply a skin barrier and verify correct sizing of the appliance.
A skin barrier will protect the damaged skin from the adhesive of the appliance, and ensuring that the appliance is not cut too large will allow for a good fit. A proper seal and fit prevent stool from collecting on the skin surface, which could create further breakdown. Changing the appliance frequently would further irritate the excoriated skin, causing trauma each time the adhesive backing was removed. Emptying the ostomy bag infrequently would increase the risk of stool overfilling the bag and pooling against the skin surrounding the ostomy. This would further irritate the already-excoriated skin. Removing the appliance and placing a dressing would not allow for collection of fecal material. It would then pool on the skin under the dressing as it is expelled, creating more damage to the skin.

119. A) Atonic seizure.
Atonic seizures are known by their loss of muscle tone and activity. Atonic seizures often cause falls due to the patient's loss of motor function. An aura is not seizure activity but is a warning sensation some patients experience prior to seizure activity or migraines. A clonic seizure is marked by rhythmic contraction and relaxation of the muscles, and a myoclonic seizure is characterized by transient jerking or stiffening of muscles; neither type of seizure is characterized by loss of muscle tone.

120. C) Decorticate posture.
Decorticate posture is indicative of brain injury and presents as extended legs with toes pointed downward and arms and hands bent in toward the body with elbows and wrists flexed. Clonus is a movement resulting from muscle contractions that appears as rapid, jerking motions and is associated with some types of seizures. While decerebrate posture results from severe injury to the brainstem, it presents as stiff extension of the legs and arms with the hands pronating outward at the wrist. Tripod positioning is noted when the patient is sitting bent forward with the arms held forward, supporting their upper body. This position is often seen in patients with respiratory impairment.

121. D) Glycated hemoglobin (glycohemoglobin A1C) 5.3% (53 g/L).
The A1C measures glycemic control over a 120-day period by measuring the reaction of glucose to hemoglobin through the erythrocytes' 120-day life cycle. The test is used both to screen for diabetes and to assess its management. This patient is showing a normal value for A1C, which is below 5.7% (57 g/L). The BUN and calcium are within normal limits, but they are not indicators of glycemic control for a patient with diabetes. Although the fasting blood glucose is high, it indicates only the current level, not the longer-term control of the patient's blood sugar.

122. B) Ask the patient whether they would like a family meeting with the provider to discuss goals of care.
The patient is expressing their psychosocial needs in relation to their physical diagnosis. It is imperative for the nurse to let the provider know and to coordinate with the patient a discussion on further interventions or goals of care. Neither pain medication as needed nor a nap addresses the patient's psychosocial need. Telling the patient they need a positive attitude is minimizing and ignoring the patient's serious concern.

123. C) Consult with case management to arrange home medication assistance on discharge.

The patient lives alone and has been unable to see the markings on the syringes. Therefore, the patient needs additional support to accurately self-administer insulin. The patient will need home health support upon discharge. Although diet is important, it is not relevant to insulin administration, which is a priority for this patient because they are insulin dependent. Because the patient is insulin dependent, an oral agent would not be indicated. Additional education is not needed because the patient is aware of insulin compliance but cannot see the syringe markings.

124. D) Open-ended questions.

Open-ended questions are used to elicit the patient's personal feelings or descriptions, known as *subjective data*. Inference is when the interviewer draws conclusions, which may or may not be correct, based on something the patient has said or the interviewer has observed. This is generally discouraged because it can lead to assumptions that are incorrect. The laundry list technique is used when the interviewer provides the patient with a list of options or terms from which the patient can choose to describe something or answer a question. This does not allow for complete subjective response from the patient. Leading questions are also to be avoided because they steer the patient toward a response that may or may not be true versus allowing the patient to respond independently.

125. A) Corticosteroids

Corticosteroids alter the body's wound healing by inhibiting the immune response and inflammation that signals for cell repair. They also cause fluid retention, which alters fluid and electrolyte balance. Insulins help control blood sugar, which improves the body's wound healing. Insulins are also important in electrolyte balance—specifically, potassium, magnesium, and phosphate. Thyroid medications are helpful to regulate appropriate amounts of thyroid hormone, which is important for wound healing. Some vitamins actually increase wound healing, such as vitamin E, and can be helpful if given postoperatively.

126. C) Rephrasing.

Rephrasing or restating the patient's response allows the patient to reflect on the response given and to clarify or verify the nurse's interpretation of the initial response. Active listening is an important part of the patient interview and helps to build trust and rapport because the listener is engaged in the patient's responses. However, it does not specifically allow for clarification of previously stated responses. Nonverbal communication is another key component of the patient interview. It helps the listener ensure that they appear interested and engaged in what the patient is saying, which builds rapport. Again, this communication technique does not allow for any clarification by the patient of previously stated responses. Silence is a nonverbal tactic used to allow time for thought or reflection. It does not specifically elicit clarification or further details of a patient's previous response.

127. B) Diabetes mellitus.
The presence of a nonhealing wound, as indicated by bandaging a cut for 2 months, indicates impaired wound healing, a complication of diabetes mellitus. Alzheimer's disease is marked by progressive cognitive decline and loss of memory and function over time. Although falls may occur in patients with Alzheimer's disease, this patient reports their recent health status and the interventions they have been taking to address the wound, which are not indicative of cognitive decline. Herpes zoster (shingles) causes a rash with weeping and crusting lesions, typically found on one laterality of the trunk along dermatomal lines. The typical duration is 3 to 5 weeks. It does not present as a nonhealing lower leg wound following an injury. Seizures occur due to abnormal electrical activity within the brain. Although they may contribute to falls, they do not correlate to delayed wound healing as experienced by this patient.

128. C) Sodium
Hyponatremia is low sodium. The nurse should monitor the serum sodium level to evaluate the patient's response to treatment. Disease processes that impact the kidneys' ability to filter and excrete, adrenal insufficiency, and certain medications can cause low sodium. Low serum sodium can lead to neurologic changes and seizures if not managed appropriately. Serum potassium is monitored for hypokalemia and hyperkalemia, which can cause dysrhythmias. Serum calcium would be monitored for hypercalcemia and hypocalcemia. Vitamin K intake should be monitored when patients are taking anticoagulant medications.

129. C) "Do you have a plan to harm yourself?"
The nurse should inquire about the patient's plan to assess risk for immediate harm. The patient may not know why they are trying to harm themselves; the nurse should inquire about suicide plans and lethality rather than the reasons behind them. The nurse should not assume or project feelings onto the patient; instead, the nurse should use therapeutic communication techniques to identify the patient's current risk of suicide. It should not be assumed that the patient uses cutting as an approach to suicide; the nurse should employ therapeutic communication techniques to identify whether the patient has a suicide plan.

130. D) Push furosemide 40 mg intravenously.
For patients experiencing congestive heart failure, the nurse should expect to administer medications that remove excess fluid from the body. Loop diuretics, such as furosemide, target the loop of Henle and inhibit the reabsorption of sodium and chloride. Administration of 0.9% normal saline at 100 mL/hr increases volume and pressure on the heart. This makes the heart work harder and perpetuates weakening of the heart. The goal of dietary therapy is to decrease the workload of the heart by decreasing sodium and water retention. Patients diagnosed with congestive heart failure should limit fluid intake to no more than 2 L/day.

131. C) Morse scale.
The Morse fall scale is used to identify patients' likelihood of falling. The Braden scale measures the likelihood of developing a pressure injury. The Glasgow Coma Scale is used to assess patients' neurologic status. The Wong–Baker FACES Scale is used to assess pain in patients.

132. A) Decrease the height of the bed to the lowest position.

Prior to and after all interactions, the nurse should ensure that the patient's environment is safe. Decreasing the height of the bed to the lowest position reduces the risk of falls in all populations. Elevating all four side rails is considered a restraint and could increase the risk for falls. When staff are not providing care, both side rails at the head of the bed should remain up to reduce the risk for falls; staff can temporarily lower a rail at the head when providing care from the same side. Removing personal items from the bedside table increases the patient's risk of falling because patients are more likely to exit the bed to retrieve them. Bed alarms are communication systems used to prevent falls; unplugging the bed alarm alters the communication system and may result in patient falls.

133. B) Obtain a stool sample.

The nurse should request an order for a stool sample. Although vancomycin (Vancocin) can be used in the treatment of *Clostridium difficile*, it can also contribute to development of that infection when used in the treatment of other disorders. The nurse should place the patient on contact precautions, wash hands with soap and water, and obtain a stool sample. Increasing the vancomycin dose could potentiate current symptoms and increase the risk of developing toxicity. Although intravenous fluids can provide hydration for lost fluid, this is not the priority recommendation. An antidiarrheal may stop diarrhea, but it does not treat the potential cause, which is infection related.

134. C) Serum potassium 5.5 mEq/L

Expected serum potassium levels are 3.5 to 5.0 mEq/L. A level of 5.5 mEq/L would be out of range. A result of 9.2 mg/dL for serum calcium is within the expected range of 9.0 to 10.5 mg/dL. The patient's serum magnesium of 2.0 mEq/L is within the expected range of 1.8 to 2.6 mEq/L. The expected range for serum sodium is 136 to 145 mEq/L.

135. D) A sharps container is located on the wall near the door entry.

A sharps container located on the wall near the door entry poses a threat to safety of a patient on suicide precautions. The nurse should remove the sharps container from the patient's room and place it in a secure place, inaccessible to the patient. Nonescape windows prevent patients on suicide precautions from harming themselves or escaping. Healthcare sitters monitor patients' actions around the clock, preventing patient self-harm. Patients on suicide precautions should not be given objects that can be used to inflict self-harm; instead, the nurse should help the patient choose food options that do not require the use of utensils, such as a sandwich. Removing plastic utensils prevents harm and does not pose a risk to the patient's safety.

136. B) Kidney

The serum creatinine level is an indicator of how well the kidneys are functioning. Blood samples can measure cardiac-specific lab values such as brain natriuretic peptide and cardiac enzymes. The use of echocardiogram can also show how well the heart is functioning. Pulmonary function tests can be used to evaluate the lungs' level of function. Assessment of a blood smear, complete blood count, and imaging studies can be used to evaluate how well the spleen is functioning.

137. A) Give the patient a blanket to fold.
A patient with dementia may fidget with different items, so the nurse can give the patient a blanket to fold. This approach can redirect the patient's attention to a safe activity. Other safe divergent activities could include arts and crafts or puzzle assembly, both in a supervised environment. Locking the patient in a quiet room alone is not appropriate; it isolates the patient and poses a safety risk. Mitts are a form of restraint; quick-release knots are used to apply wrist restraints to a nonmovable part of the bedframe. Neither would be appropriate when seeking restraint alternatives.

138. C) Intravenously push an amp of 50% dextrose (D50).
The nurse understands that the patient is experiencing a hypoglycemic event as evidenced by diaphoretic appearance, change in mentation, and low blood glucose reading. The nurse should administer 50% dextrose (D50) via intravenous push route to increase the circulation of glucose in the bloodstream. Administering five units of rapid-acting insulin will decrease the blood glucose level further. Conducting an in-depth neurologic assessment prolongs glucose deprivation. The patient appears diaphoretic because of the cholinergic response; placing a cool, damp towel on the patient's forehead does not address the low blood glucose level.

139. B) Apply airborne precaution personal protective equipment.
The patient presents with classic signs of tuberculosis. To prevent the potential spread of infection, the nurse will apply airborne precaution personal protective equipment before caring for the patient. The nurse should obtain a sputum culture prior to the administration of antibiotics because drugs could alter the culture and sensitivity report. If a provider orders thoracentesis, it will occur only after precautions are in place; additionally, the provider is responsible for obtaining consent. Similarly, although obtaining a sputum culture may be necessary for the patient's treatment plan, it would occur only after protective measures are in place.

140. A) Fell at home 1 month ago.
Extra safety precautions would be put in place for the patient who fell at home 1 month ago. A previous fall is the single biggest indicator for future falls. The nurse should use evidence-based fall-prevention interventions to keep the patient safe while in the hospital. An asthma diagnosis does not increase the patient's risk for falls. Nonskid shoes reduce the risk for falls during ambulation. The use of a wheelchair does not predict the patient's likelihood of falling.

141. A) Assess the peripheral pulses.
The nurse should assess the patient's peripheral pulses to ensure that there is adequate perfusion. The nurse should not keep the patient in a supine position because this can lead to aspiration and choking. The nurse should elevate the head of the bed to at least 30 to 45 degrees. Keeping the patient NPO can lead to dehydration and compromise skin integrity. The nurse should offer the patient food and fluids throughout the shift. Tying the restraints to the bedrails can cause injury; the nurse should tie a quick-release knot to a nonmovable part of the bedframe.

142. B) Gown.

Methicillin-resistant *Staphylococcus aureus* in wounds is transferred by direct contact with the contaminant; therefore, the nurse should apply a gown and gloves prior to performing wound care. It is not necessary for the nurse to apply a face shield. A surgical mask is used for droplet precautions, but it is not necessary for patients with methicillin-resistant *Staphylococcus aureus* in a wound. An N95 respirator should be applied when caring for patients on airborne precautions.

143. D) Let the provider know the patient may need depression screening.

The patient may be experiencing situational depression due to the recent diagnosis, and the provider needs to be notified for a more formal screening and medical diagnosis so interventions may occur. The patient is not stating that pain is a current issue, so pain medication would not be administered. Chiding the patient for expressing their feelings is inappropriate, and suggesting that rest will improve their feelings ignores the potential seriousness of the situation.

144. D) Surgical mask, gown, and gloves.

Given the patient's age, university attendance, and symptoms, the nurse should suspect bacterial meningitis. The nurse needs to apply a surgical mask, gown, and gloves to prevent transmission, which occurs by oral and respiratory droplets. A face shield will not protect against droplet transmission. An N95 respirator is unnecessary because it is intended for airborne-transmitted contaminants. Nurses should preserve equipment for appropriate use, preventing waste and supporting cost containment.

145. B) Suspect hospital delirium and incorporate interventions.

The patient has been in the ICU for 10 days, and hallucinations and disorientation are hallmarks of ICU delirium. The nurse would reorient the patient, assess for pain, assist the patient with mobilization, and encourage adequate hydration, nutrition, and elimination patterns. Letting the patient sleep all day will exacerbate delirium symptoms. Telling the patient that there are no bugs in the room or asking the spouse to stay in the room will not address the delirium.

146. B) Educate the patient that this medication only assists with symptoms.

There is no cure for Parkinson's disease. Carbidopa and levodopa (Sinemet) treatment helps with neurologic symptoms. Medication education is not successful as long as the patient incorrectly believes the drug will cure the disease. Carbidopa and levodopa must be taken daily to adequately manage the neurologic symptoms of Parkinson's disease. Telling the patient they should not be so confident is not therapeutic communication.

147. D) Use the Pain Assessment in Advanced Dementia (PAINAD) scale for observational assessment.

The patient has dementia, and the proper tool to use is the PAINAD scale. The patient will not accurately be able to state a number or react to faces because they are disoriented. Documenting "no pain" is inaccurate based on the patient's cognitive level. Pain needs to be assessed, and using the appropriate pain scale is necessary.

148. B) Has short-term memory issues and needs frequent reorientation.
A patient who has just completed breakfast and then asks when the meal will occur is most likely experiencing short-term memory loss, and the nurse would further assess the patient's short-term memory. Short-term memory loss is not being able to recall something within 60 minutes, and these patients need frequent reorientation and visual cues. Because the patient is asking about breakfast rather than asking for more food, it is more likely that they have forgotten that the meal was just served than that the patient remembers the meal but is still hungry. The patient's question does not indicate that they are experiencing a stroke or exhibiting signs of low blood sugar.

149. C) Ineffective airway clearance.
When prioritizing nursing diagnoses, airway is the first priority, then breathing, followed by circulation. Risk for inadequate nutrition is the lowest priority.

150. D) Ask whether the patient has ever been assessed for attention deficit disorder (ADD).
The patient is exhibiting criteria for ADD. The nurse should inquire whether the patient has ever been assessed for ADD and arrange a consult with the appropriate provider. Telling the patient to calm down is not therapeutic communication and is not helpful to the patient. Asking the patient about job status is irrelevant to the patient's symptoms, and a physical assessment is not the immediate concern for this patient.